THE
MILLENNIAL
CAREGIVER

THE MILLENNIAL CAREGIVER

Caring for Loved Ones in the Busiest Years of Your Life

RACHAEL PILTCH-LOEB

SUTHERLAND HOUSE

TORONTO, 2025

Sutherland House
416 Moore Ave., Suite 304
Toronto, ON M4G 1C9

First edition, March 2025

If you are interested in inviting one of our authors to a live event or
media appearance, please contact sranasinghe@sutherlandhousebooks.com
and visit our website at sutherlandhousebooks.com for more information.

We acknowledge the support of the Government of Canada.

Manufactured in China
Cover designed by Lena Yang and Leah Ciani
Book composed by Karl Hunt

Library and Archives Canada Cataloguing in Publication
Title: The millennial caregiver : caring for loved ones in the busiest
years of your life / Rachael Piltch-Loeb, PhD, MSPH.
Names: Piltch-Loeb, Rachael, author.
Description: Includes bibliographical references.
Identifiers: Canadiana (print) 20240519345 | Canadiana (ebook) 2024051937X
| ISBN 9781998365197 (softcover) | ISBN 9781998365203 (EPUB)
Subjects: LCSH: Caregivers. | LCSH: Generation Y. |
LCSH: Aging parents—Care. | LCSH: Care of the sick.
Classification: LCC RA645.3 .P55 2025 | DDC 362.14—dc23

ISBN 978-1-998365-19-7
eBook 978-1-998365-20-3

CONTENTS

Chapter 1: Introduction   1

Chapter 2: Understanding the Millennial Caregiver   14

Chapter 3: Planning   24

Chapter 4: Balancing   39

Chapter 5: Effective Communication and Family Dynamics   52

Chapter 6: Healthcare Management and Advocacy   67

Chapter 7: Digital Tools   81

Chapter 8: Financial Realities   96

Chapter 9: Career Development   110

Chapter 10: Coping with Grief and Loss   125

Appendix 1: Long-Term Illness Care Planning Template   137

Appendix 2: Re-evaluation Care Planning Template   142

*Chapter 4: Appendix: The CALMER Steps to Balancing
Caregiving Responsibility*   145

Chapter 8: Appendix: Financial Budget Worksheet   147

Notes   150

CHAPTER 1

Introduction

CAREGIVING IS HARD. CAREGIVING FOR SOMEONE with a terminal illness can be even harder. Add on top of that trying to be a young adult, learning to parent, advance professionally, save money, and have a social life, and you have what can feel like an overwhelming burden. I know. I've been there.

My journey as a caregiver was characterized by a striking dichotomy: my first child was born as my dad was diagnosed with Alzheimer's disease. As I was supporting a baby—later a toddler—as it learned the world around it, I was also watching my father—a strong, happy, capable man—regress and navigate the shrinking reality that comes with cognitive decline. As I shared my journey with people I cared about, it was hard to put into words. It still is. But it's the dichotomy of happiness and sadness, living and losing. Watching my father deal with cognitive decline was parenting without the bright horizon, the knowledge that with enough positive reinforcement, a task will get mastered, and a person will grow. We would often joke that he had the easiest time hanging with his grandson, the toddler, because they had similar mental capacities. It became dark humor the more the toddler learned and Dad forgot.

Sometimes when Dad was sick, my mom and I would commiserate. We were each dealing with temper tantrums. Hers were when Dad wanted to drive and didn't understand why he couldn't, so he was throwing the keys and threatening to get in the car, or grabbing the steering wheel while she was driving. Mine were when my son wanted to have a toy that he couldn't have and threw his food on the floor in protest. We laughed. More dark humor. But the undertone was starkly different. There was hope—there is still hope!—that my toddler will grow out of this phase. Dad, on the other hand, was going to move on from this phase: he was going to forget what driving was altogether, or that driving was an activity he was once able to do.

Dad was an excellent driver. Or at least that's how I remember it. He taught me how to drive when I got my learner's permit. He sacrificed his truck a couple of times and dutifully banged out the dents when I took a turn too tight. One of my first losses when his memory started to fade was that I could no longer call him for directions. Dad always had a specific opinion on how to get from the home where my parents raised us to his parents' home, a few states away. Each time I drove that route as an adult, I would call to confirm which parkway to take. Each time, he would carefully instruct me. I remember my first drive after his dementia set in. I called as usual. I asked him to confirm the exit number and the parkway name, and his voice trailed off. There was silence, and a mumbled "yeah." I was confused and missed the turn.

The only consequence was an extra half hour of traffic, but it was a major reminder that my life was going to change as my dad changed. A couple of months later, I repeated the drive. By then, I had moved to the same city as my grandparents and would commute back to see my parents at regular intervals. When I got to my parents' house, my dad was out of it. He was sitting in a chair in the garden and got up to say hello when I arrived. I walked him through the steps I took to get home, elated because I knew I had followed his directions. I hoped that the names of the streets I mentioned would jog his memory, but they didn't. He said "great," he was glad I was there, and moved on. We didn't get to banter about the most efficient route and those unlucky others who drove the traditional way. Dad was no longer the bantering type. Another little moment that said things were changing.

One of the things that struck me most about my dad's decline was that I noticed it in these little moments. Small things that I had come to rely upon changed. They would never be the same. In her eulogy after my dad died, my sister reflected that this was the hardest part. Our dad was not a man for grand gestures or milestones. He was consistent. He showed up each day with a clear head and even temperament. He rarely got irritated. In fact, I can count on one hand the two times in childhood he lost his cool—once at a remote control when my younger brother and I wouldn't stop fighting; the other at a dishwasher that simply stopped working. He took things one step at a time, day after day. He taught us to be present and focus on the little things.

That's why we found the small changes problematic. We were acutely aware that something was off when Dad stopped being able to do mental math. This was a man who had decided at age fifty he was done with his career as a general contractor; he wanted to get a degree in education and become a middle school math teacher. Who in their right mind volunteers to teach math or hang out with middle schoolers? My dad!

As his dementia advanced, he once fell asleep at the wheel. Another time, he got lost on his way home. My sister was in the car, and he laughed it off, saying he was just tired. An avid crossword player his entire life, he was now having trouble finding words. My mom discovered bills had gone unpaid and that he had a couple of new credit cards. When he lost one, he would sign up for another card rather than replacing it. These little changes led dad to a series of doctors who conducted neurologic and cognitive testing over the course of several months. While his official diagnosis was prolonged by pandemic-era delays to non-emergency healthcare services, the prognosis, when it finally came, was unequivocal. Dad had early-onset Alzheimer's and was expected to live no more than five years. He was fifty-eight.

When Alzheimer's disease occurs in someone under age sixty-five, it is known as early-onset (or younger-onset) Alzheimer's disease. A very small number of people with Alzheimer's disease have the early-onset form. Many of them are in their forties and fifties when the disease takes hold.[1] According to a 2021 meta-analysis, the global age-standardized prevalence of young-onset dementia was 119 per 100,000 population, or approximately 1 in 1,000 people in the world.[2] Only 5 to 6 percent of people with Alzheimer's will develop symptoms before the age of sixty-five. My dad happened to be one of them.

Alzheimer's disease typically occurs in four phases: pre-clinical, when protein is building in the brain (this is before symptoms typically start); mild, when some of those small changes are noticeable (there may be trouble paying bills or forgetfulness); moderate, characterized by difficulty with language, trouble learning new things, and sometimes changes in mood or temperament; and advanced, an inability to communicate, changes to sleep, inability to do the functions of daily living. Critically, Alzheimer's may not be characterized by forgetting people. Dad always seemed to register who we were. He just lost many other abilities. How quickly each phase comes is dependent on a case-by-case basis, but for those who are diagnosed younger, the trajectory is often more rapid. From the time of diagnosis to death, my dad lived less than three years.

What was surprising about Dad's diagnosis and decline was that he was so able-bodied. When you looked at him, he was slim, his slightly olive skin was tanned, his hair salt and pepper, and he was active. He played basketball and tennis, went biking, enjoyed going for walks, and attempted to golf. He was the picture of health. But the picture was not reality. I remember talking to a close friend after her parents told her that her dad was dying of amyotrophic lateral sclerosis (ALS), Lou Gehrig's disease, another neurodegenerative condition that has escaped our medical understanding. My friend and her siblings had noticed that their incredibly active father—jet-skiing, skydiving, golfing, boating, tubing, etc.—was having back problems. Her parents had initially said that he needed back surgery. This went on for nearly a year until the day of the alleged surgery. The siblings were brought together and told it was not just a back condition but a degenerative diagnosis with a poor prognosis. The picture of health had allowed the family one extra year of perceived normalcy. The siblings got to continue with their schooling and careers while their parents coped with the diagnosis in secret. Looks can be deceiving.

Caregiving is a very personal experience. I luckily had a spouse who was always there to listen, but when friends would ask how my dad was doing, I never knew what to say. Did they really want to know? He wasn't doing well. How could he be doing well? His brain wasn't working normally, and he was never going to get better. That's not to say I didn't appreciate people thinking about me, or him, or our family. I most certainly did. But I found it incredibly hard to share my experience even with my closest friends. Without being in my position, it was nearly impossible for someone to understand how challenging these times were. It took too much energy to explain the daily difficulties, to really try to make someone understand. I found support groups, primarily through Zoom, to be a somewhat helpful venting ground, but the frequency and consistency of the groups was limited. Many of the other participants were not my age. Most people with a parent ailing from Alzheimer's were much older. I often felt isolated in my coping.

This was a theme in my search for support. When I looked for resources as I became a caregiver, and for a support system to another caregiver (my mom), everything I found was geared toward seniors. My dad wasn't a senior. He'd never seemed old. Still in his fifties and able-bodied, he wasn't frail. His kids were young; my siblings hadn't finished school or married. We had to come to terms with the fact that Dad wasn't going to be there for the many things we had envisioned him being a part of. And we had to learn how to be caregivers ourselves.

My family's experience caring for my dad was the inspiration for this book. There were so many things that we had to do, not only to support Dad, but to make sure we sustained our own lives. Caregiving is a constant slog of day-to-day tasks. And while you are focused on the day-to-day decisions—what therapy may help stave off the next stage of disease, if even for a brief amount of time, or which shower bar will offer the most support without cracking the tiles on your 100-year-old bathroom wall when pulled on by a large man with a mobility issue—the big changes happen. For me, those big changes included becoming a parent. For my brother, it was getting married and buying his first home. For my sister, it was finding her career passion and completing her degree. We each achieved different life milestones while struggling to support our mom and be a caregiving team to our dad.

Being young and coping with caregiving is a growing phenomenon. According to a report by AARP, as of 2020, approximately 24 percent of caregivers in the United States are millennials (then defined as eighteen to thirty-four). This proportion is expected to increase as the baby boomer generation ages. Millennial caregivers, now in their late twenties to early forties, face distinct challenges: they are looking after loved ones while simultaneously building their careers and starting families. This was obvious to me when I became a millennial caregiver, but it was helpful to have some facts to back up what I was feeling. Millennials, like me, are a distinct generation in their information consumption behavior, family dynamics, employment status, and mental health needs. We are digital natives and are more likely to rely on technology and digital tools to aid in caregiving responsibilities. One survey found that 91 percent of millennial caregivers use technology to manage caregiving tasks, such as researching health information, scheduling appointments, and coordinating care with other family members or healthcare professionals. Another found that 34 percent of millennial caregivers are simultaneously caring for children under the age of eighteen and an ailing parent. This dual responsibility of caregiving for both older adults and children places additional demands on time and resources.

Given the number of millennial caregivers out there in the population, I knew my experience could not be unique. There were thousands of other people going through caregiving as young adults. So, I put my professional skills to work and started researching what being a young adult caregiver looked like. I had spent over a decade in higher education, trained as a research scientist—this was my home-run derby. I pored over the literature on caregiving norms, interventions, and support strategies. There weren't many tailored toward young people *at all*.

I learned a few things about what made caregiving at a younger age particularly challenging:

- Role Reversal: taking on caregiver responsibilities for an aging parent at a younger age can feel like a significant role reversal. Fundamentally, you are used to being cared for by your parent. That changes drastically. It is emotionally challenging to see a parent who was once strong and independent now in need of care.
- Balancing Life Transitions and Multiple Roles: the nature of being young(er) means that you are likely in a chronic

transitional phase. Maybe you are still searching for a home of your own, a partner, or starting a career or family. Younger caregivers often find themselves balancing these transitions with caregiving responsibilities. This juggling act can be overwhelming, as they must divide their time and energy among various roles, often experiencing feelings of guilt and self-doubt.

- Limited Life Experience: Younger caregivers may have less experience to draw on than their older counterparts. They may not have as much knowledge about medical conditions, navigating healthcare systems, or complex caregiving situations. Younger generations tend to be less connected to in-person healthcare facilities, preferring online modalities to access care. This lack of experience can add an extra layer of stress and a steeper learning curve in patient navigation on behalf of someone else.

- Impact on Personal Relationships: caring for a parent at a younger age can affect personal relationships. It may require understanding and support from partners, friends, or other family members, who may not have anticipated taking on caregiving responsibilities at this stage of life, and who may be as ill-equipped to take on this supporting role. Maintaining open communication and seeking assistance from loved ones can be crucial in managing these dynamics. Asking for that kind of help is hard.

- Emotional and Psychological Impact: caregiving can take a toll on millennials' emotional and psychological well-being. Witnessing the physical and cognitive decline of a loved one, managing medical crises, and making difficult decisions about healthcare can be emotionally draining. Caregiver burnout, stress, anxiety, and depression are common challenges that all caregivers face, especially when they struggle to prioritize their own self-care needs.

- Social Isolation: younger caregivers may face a generational gap between themselves and other caregivers. Younger caregivers may not find as many peers going through a similar experience, which can make it harder to find support, share experiences, and seek guidance from those who can relate. It is also natural in our current society to compare your own life to that of others, and the life of a caregiver is often far from glamorous. This can contribute to feelings of loneliness and envy.

- Financial Considerations: younger caregivers may face financial challenges unique to their age group. They may still be paying off student loans, starting to build their savings, or establishing their careers. Balancing caregiving expenses with personal financial goals can be difficult and may require creative financial planning or seeking assistance from available resources. Taking on caregiving responsibilities can further strain their finances, as they may need to cover expenses related to medical care, home modifications, and additional support services. The financial burden can lead to increased stress and limited resources for their own personal and professional goals.

- Limited Workplace Support: Millennials often encounter workplace challenges that hinder their caregiving responsibilities. Many face inflexible work hours, lack of paid leave, and limited understanding from employers about the demands of caregiving. This can lead to conflicts between work and caregiving responsibilities, forcing millennials to make difficult choices and potentially impacting career growth, and, in turn, financial stability.

- Caregiving Complexities: millennials may find it challenging to access adequate resources and support services for caregiving. Affordable healthcare options, respite care, and professional assistance can be limited, leaving younger caregivers to navigate the complexities of caregiving on their own. The lack of community support and awareness about millennial caregivers' unique needs can further compound their challenges. There are very

limited resources that provide guidance on the all-encompassing
nature of caregiving, let alone how to balance that with all of the
other complexities of life.

- Impact on Future Plans: as a younger caregiver, the responsibility of caring for a parent can impact future plans and personal
goals. It may require adjusting career aspirations, delaying educational pursuits, or altering lifestyle choices. Considering the
long-term implications and making decisions that align with
personal and caregiving needs can be complex and require careful thought. Many millennial caregivers face the daunting task
of planning for their own long-term future while providing care.
They must balance their current caregiving responsibilities with
concerns about their own financial security, retirement savings,
and future care needs. The uncertainty of their own caregiving
journey can add additional stress and anxiety.

I have spent my entire thirties learning to be a mom, a professional,
and a caregiver. There are few things in life as disruptive as becoming a parent and losing a parent. In both instances, you become a
new version of yourself. You are forced to grow, mature, and change
because the person who existed before no longer has the same time,
the same foundation, and the same mindset. I experienced both
changes over the course of three years.

This book is a result of my research and my experience. The
research was my way of coping with a declining and demoralizing
situation. The stories are all true and all personal. When I refer to a
friend or family member, I have asked their permission to share their
story. Through this book, you will find a tailored look at caregiving
as a millennial. Although my experience was caring for a parent with
a neurodegenerative condition, almost all of the takeaways apply if
you are caring for a spouse or a sibling or another loved one, or if the
disease you are dealing with is cancer or heart disease or something

else entirely. Many of the burdens associated with being a person and a caregiver are universal. The book focuses on how to address the specific situations and concerns that our generation faces when caregiving. By providing relatable examples and scenarios, the book supports millennial caregivers in their experience. A few things you will find in this book:

- A Focus on Work–Life Integration: being a caregiver and showing up to work every day is a task. Caregiving is a job. Many people do it professionally! But when you are in the throes of being a part-time caregiver and full-time professional, you are rarely fully present. Finding balance is hard. Because younger adults tend to be at earlier stages of their career, achieving work–life balance and integrating caregiving responsibilities with career aspirations is especially challenging. This book can provide insights and strategies for managing time, setting boundaries, and communicating with employers about caregiving needs. It will also explore flexible work arrangements, caregiving leave policies, and resources for career development while balancing caregiving responsibilities.

- A Description of Health and Digital Resources: Google has been a good friend to me throughout my search for answers on my dad's disease. I would research his new medication regimes, therapies that may help him, and pretty much anything else. Digital tools can be a huge help in research, organization, and advocacy, but they can also be daunting. Younger caregivers, by nature, are generally tech-savvy (maybe some more than me?), and a caregiving book for our generation must explore the role of technology in caregiving. This book will highlight useful online resources and support networks available to assist millennial caregivers in managing their responsibilities effectively.

Additionally, this book can offer guidance on utilizing digital tools for communication, healthcare management, and coordination with other caregivers or healthcare professionals.

- A Discussion of Financial Considerations: it's hard to think about paying for caregiving, or pitching in, when your own financial future is uncertain. Many younger caregivers face financial challenges such as student loan debt, housing costs, and saving for the future. Even though some younger caregivers may not be solely responsible for caregiving costs, it's important to recognize just how many hidden costs there are to dealing with a terminal illness and try to get ahead of as many of these as possible. This book will touch on the financial aspects of caregiving, including budgeting, accessing financial assistance programs, understanding insurance options, and planning for retirement while managing caregiving responsibilities. It can provide practical strategies for navigating these financial hurdles and attempting to maintain financial well-being.

- Attention to Mental Health and Self-care: pretty much any free mental space can become occupied by the emotional toll of coping with caregiving. There is the day-to-day stress of appointments, changing relationships, family dynamics, and just living. There is the anticipatory grief of knowing someone is dying. Sometimes there is guilt when you have fun, but you know that your loved one won't be able to participate. All of these emotions are burdensome and conflicting and can take their toll. Millennial caregivers may encounter increased stress and mental health challenges due to the juggling of multiple roles and responsibilities. As a younger adult, you still want to have fun and enjoy life, and sometimes that is hard! This tailored caregiving book will emphasize the importance of self-care and offer specific self-care strategies that resonate with millennials and support personal growth in the caregiving process. It will include topics like mindfulness, stress reduction techniques, seeking therapy or counseling, and finding peer-support networks specifically designed for millennial caregivers.

- Ways to Find Social Connections and Community Support: finding social support while coping as a caregiver can be especially challenging. There is the constant debate over whether to share or not share what you are going through. There is the desire to connect, but the exhaustion of the situation. Generally, millennials value community and connections, both online and offline. This book includes guidance on building support networks, connecting with other millennial caregivers through online communities or social media, and finding local resources or support groups. It describes the importance of social connections and offers strategies for maintaining relationships while fulfilling caregiving responsibilities.

- Within these pages you will also find tools like websites and apps that may be helpful for caregiving, a care plan template, sample scripts for working through caregiving responsibilities with other family members, and lots of anecdotes.

I learned so much over the past few years—my whole family has—about how to be a caregiver, a daughter, a sibling, a parent, a spouse, and a friend. I felt like I could have used a resource like this, and I hope it can help someone else.

CHAPTER 2

Understanding the Millennial Caregiver

'M NOT SURE I WAS EVER CLEAR ON WHAT DEFINED my generation until I started reading up on what it means to be a Millennial. I felt seen. I most definitely favor Instagram over TikTok, prefer reading about things online before going to explore them in person, and I love e-commerce. I scoff at Gen Z and its obsession with TikTok, despite admitting that I am totally behind the times and end up re-watching TikToks when they get posted two weeks later to Instagram. I know some slang but definitely not the latest trends. I've at times embraced the coastal grandma trend associated with Nancy Meyers' movies. I held on to my Blackberry for too long because I was convinced touch screens would not work for me. I am a classic Millennial.

Being a millennial has been a defining factor in my caregiving experience. I belong to a generation that is part of what I would like to call "the new sandwich generation." The original sandwich generation referred to middle-aged adults (perhaps in their forties or fifties, caring for their own children and their elderly parents. The new sandwich generation has aging but not conventionally old parents. Many of our grandparents may still be alive. We have youngish kids, or maybe we're thinking about having kids. That means there are more sandwich layers above us than below us. That means there are many different interpersonal relationships to navigate, especially in caregiving. Also that there may be multiple people who need care in different ways.

My experience of being a young parent and dealing with my not old father being sick and then dying has defined a lot of my life in my thirties. My friends who have also watched a parent ail know it can be all-consuming. It feels premature to experience their death. It feels unfair. There are still so many milestones that we expect our parents to be part of that it seems to go against nature. And yet, it happens. Though the average life expectancy in the United States and Canada is now seventies and eighties, many older adults are living with chronic, debilitating conditions much earlier.

This chapter will be brief, but it explains a bit about millennials and why there is a need for a whole book about what it means to be both a millennial and a caregiver, and, more importantly, how to take those generation-defining characteristics and adapt.

Characterizing Millennials

The millennial generation, also known as Generation Y, refers to the cohort of individuals born roughly between the early 1980s and the mid-1990s. While there is no universally agreed-upon definition, millennials tended to be in grade school or secondary school on September 11, 2001, a day that forever changed perceptions of safety and security and global politics. Millennials were young workers or professionals, working on establishing careers or entering parenthood when the COVID-19 pandemic hit, disrupting ways of life, some of which were forever changed. Perhaps most unique to millennials is being the cohort that has grown up with digital technology.

As a millennial, you remember your first computer, your first cellphone, and the various devices that have defined life. Who can't recall the leap from waiting for your mom to finish a call on the family landline to coming home and being able to chat with friends instantly over AOL Messenger (AIM). My siblings and I spent hours playing Oregon Trail, Carmen San Diego, and SIMS on our shared family computer. My first personal computer was an orange Mac laptop I got in high school. I only needed to type documents, and it was slow as molasses, but I felt *cool* having that thing all to myself.

Millennials have been the first generation to fully embrace and integrate digital technology into daily life. The rise of the personal computer gave way to the commonality of the internet and, in parallel, social networking sites. That integration has now become ubiquitous. Far more than previous generations, millennials use smartphones, social media, and other digital platforms for communication, information access, and entertainment. According to the Pew Research Center, 92 percent of millennials (ages twenty-three to thirty-eight at the time of the survey) own smartphones, compared to 58 percent of baby boomers (ages fifty-five to seventy-three) and 74 percent of Generation X (ages thirty-nine to fifty-four). The same study found that 85 percent of millennials use social media, compared to 48 percent of baby boomers and 77 percent of Generation X.

We're the first generation to become accustomed to having the most up-to-date information at our fingertips, the first to message our partners and expect a response in a minute (or less). Our most common platforms are X (formerly Twitter), Instagram, Reddit, and Facebook. We are steeped in our online communities, sharing experiences and opinions and engaging in social activism through digital platforms. Our expectation of constant access to information and comfort with technology also means that we expect quick answers to questions and get stressed when that is not possible. We are keenly aware of our higher levels of technological adoption and digital literacy, especially when we have to walk our able-minded mothers or fathers through new devices or platforms.

As a product of technology and connectivity, millennials are sometimes characterized as more diverse in their thinking and experiences, with increased exposure to different cultures, ethnicities, and perspectives. Globalization in business, travel, and e-commerce has created the potential for multiple identities. Millennials have been at the vanguard of such cultural issues as inclusivity, equality, and social justice. Millennials actively seek diverse environments and value representation and inclusivity in their personal and professional lives.

Compared to their parents, millennials have higher levels of educational attainment, driven by the belief that it leads to better career prospects. The US Bureau of Labor Statistics reported that in 2020, 40 percent of millennials held a bachelor's degree or higher, compared to 30 percent of baby boomers at a similar age. The National Center for Education Statistics found that 40 percent of millennials held a bachelor's degree or higher in 2019, compared to 31 percent of Generation X and 26 percent of baby boomers at the same age. However, millennials have also faced challenges in the job market, experiencing higher rates of unemployment and underemployment compared to their parents. And a study by the Pew Research Center found that millennials have experienced slower wage growth compared to previous generations at a similar age.

The Millennial pursuit of higher education has been expensive. According to the Pew Research Center, 63 percent of millennials have outstanding student loan debt, a reality that sets them apart from previous generations. This has affected their financial stability and home-ownership rates, and delayed major life decisions, such as starting families. A study by the Center for Financial Services

Innovation found that 57 percent of millennials struggle with financial health, including issues with income volatility, managing expenses, and saving for the future. The Federal Reserve Bank of St. Louis reported that 43 percent of millennials owned homes in 2020, compared to 49 percent of Generation X and 59 percent of baby boomers at similar ages. The same study reported that the median net worth of millennials in 2020 was $19,000, compared to $44,000 for Generation X and $123,000 for baby boomers. The economic challenges of Millennials have been exacerbated by the 2008 financial crisis and the recent COVID-19 pandemic, two more factors that have influenced their ability to get married, buy homes, and start families.

Millennials tend to have different professional values and attitudes compared to their parents. They often prioritize work–life balance and personal fulfillment over traditional markers of success, such as financial wealth or job stability. Deloitte's Millennial Survey 2020 revealed that 55 percent of millennials prioritize work–life balance and personal well-being as important factors when considering job opportunities. It also showed that 74 percent of Millennials believe that businesses have a positive impact on society, compared to 59 percent of Generation X and 50 percent of baby boomers. A survey by Bentley University found that 84 percent of Millennials believe it is their duty to make a positive difference in the world. A study by the IBM Institute for Business Value found that 72 percent of Millennials believe it is important for a company to have a purpose-driven mission, compared to 58 percent of Generation X and 48 percent of baby boomers. Millennials have also shown a greater inclination toward entrepreneurship and self-employment compared to previous generations. This is consistent with their appreciation of flexibility in their work arrangements, their prioritization of work–life balance, and preference for job opportunities that align with their personal values and passions.

The consumer behavior of millennials differs from their parents in several ways. They prioritize experiences over material possessions, prefer sustainable and socially responsible products, and rely heavily on online shopping. Millennials also value personalized and tailored experiences, which has influenced the rise of customization and personalization in various industries. A study by Accenture found that 62 percent of millennials prefer to spend money on experiences rather than material possessions. Nielsen reported that 73 percent of millennials are willing to pay more for sustainable products.

Millennials exhibit lower levels of political engagement and party identification than their parents do. A survey by the Pew Research Center found that they are less likely to identify as Republicans compared to older generations, with 45 percent of millennials leaning Democratic or identifying as Democrats, and 35 percent leaning Republican or identifying as Republicans. They are more likely to identify as independent or unaffiliated with political parties. However, millennials have shown active engagement in social and political issues, often using digital platforms for activism and advocacy. A study by the Harvard Kennedy School's Institute of Politics revealed that 44 percent of millennials have participated in protests or rallies.

Millennials are generally more health-conscious than their parents. They prioritize physical and mental well-being, engage in exercise and fitness activities, and seek out healthy food options. The National Center for Health Statistics reported that millennials have lower obesity rates than previous generations, with 22 percent of millennials classified as obese, compared to 32 percent of baby boomers. They are more apt to seek mental health services and acknowledge their psychological needs than older generations. They also exhibit higher levels of stress and mental health challenges, potentially attributed to various factors like financial pressures and the influence of technology. The American Psychological Association reported that 45 percent of millennials have been diagnosed with a mental health disorder, compared to 38 percent of Generation X and 21 percent of baby boomers. According to a study published in JAMA Network Open, millennials have seen a higher increase in rates of major depression compared to their parents at a similar age.

Millennials and Caregiving

Ok, you get it. Millennials have some unique traits that are a product of being born at a certain point in time. Who cares? What does all this mean for me as a caregiver?

It means a lot! Age, experience, and life state can make caregiving more or less challenging. For millennials, it means taking on the challenges of being a caregiver while you are still relatively young. In fact, you may still be in a stage of life defined as "emerging adulthood." That means you are in the long transitional period between youth, with its structured set of steps for personal and professional progression, and adulthood, where these norms and routines are more solidified and established.

One general theory about age and development called "The Life Course Health Development (LCHD) model[3]" tells us that emerging adulthood is a life stage when people experience changes along many different dimensions, including the cognitive, emotional, physical, and social. During this same period of life, people also tend to experience changes to their living environment and make choices that can be critical to long-term development. Naturally, watching the decline of a loved one, and having this stage of life disrupted by a new set of responsibilities and unknown factors, can be incredibly challenging. In other words, the period of life that you are now in is already one that includes many developmental challenges, so adding caregiving to it can be daunting and have long-term repercussions.

There are also practical challenges for millennials who become caregivers. The financial burdens mentioned earlier can impact a person's ability to provide financial support for their loved ones or to take time off work for caregiving responsibilities. It may require a delicate balance between caregiving and maintaining one's own financial stability, potentially seeking flexible work arrangements or exploring assistance programs to manage caregiving costs. Millennials are more likely to report being the sole unpaid caregiver (compared to older generations) and fewer report having paid help.[4] They more often report high levels of financial strain and financial impacts as a result of caregiving, including more debt, unpaid or late-paid bills, borrowing from friends or family, and an inability to afford basic expenses such as food.

Striking a financial and professional balance is difficult. A 2020 study found that millennials, who are typically working while providing care, were less likely to report that their supervisor at work is aware of their caregiving role, yet were more likely to have received a warning about their performance or attendance at work.[5] The pressure to succeed professionally and maintain personal well-being while fulfilling caregiving duties can lead to increased stress, and the need for smart strategies to manage time, set boundaries, and prioritize self-care.[6]

All caregivers need support from their personal networks and professional allies. For millennials, this literally means having a therapist—they rate mental health treatment as most helpful for managing stress—as well as more basic support from family and friends. That basic support can be complicated, given that millennials often have diverse family structures and caregiving dynamics compared to previous generations. They may be caring for aging parents, grandparents, siblings, or other relatives, including chosen family members—relationships that can be complex to navigate not only socially but legally and in decision-making processes.

There are also some advantages to being a millennial caregiver. For example, you are able to use your skills in digital literacy and technology to your advantage. Leveraging the tools that are part of your daily life can make caregiving a more seamless process. There are digital tools and apps and online resources for *so* many caregiving responsibilities. They make it easier to access information, coordinate care, seek support, and communicate with healthcare providers, pharmacists, and therapists. A millennial caregiver is also able to tap into telehealth services, remote monitoring devices, and communication platforms to stay connected with healthcare providers.

As mentioned earlier, millennials are also much more comfortable acknowledging their own need for mental health support, which can be critical to caregiver well-being. Millennials tend to be more proactive in seeking therapy or counseling to manage the emotional challenges. They may also prioritize self-care practices and stress reduction, understanding the importance of maintaining their own well-being while caring for others. Have you ever practiced Mindfulness? Listened to a meditation podcast? Just set aside time for exercise or a walk? Many millennials have an acknowledgment of the need for personal and mental breaks that become critical as caretaking tasks increase.

Connecting to other caregivers can help ease the feelings of isolation and frustration that may come with being a caregiver. However, there are so many electronic ways to connect with other caregivers and gather support and advice.

Because they grew up in a rapidly changing world, millennials often exhibit resourcefulness, adaptability, and a willingness to reach out. This can be very useful in seeking connections to other caregivers, a big help in alleviating the isolation and frustration that can come with the role, and a great source of support and advice. They may even be able to tap into formal caregiving resources through online searches and communities. For example, there may be home health aide websites to search or other specialized therapists to reach through social networking or professional service websites. All of this can be used to your advantage. There will always be a diversity of experiences in caregiving. Understanding generational influences can help support millennial caregivers by tailoring resources, services, and support to millennials' specific needs. Factors such as cultural background, socioeconomic status, and individual circumstances can further shape anyone's caregiving journey. Through the rest of the book, I will help you think through how to address your generation-specific needs to give your best as a caregiver.

CHAPTER 3

Planning

I CLEARLY REMEMBER THE DAY MY DAD WAS DIAGNOSED with Alzheimer's. He got the call from his doctor. His test results were back. He had a large build-up of protein in his spine; it was indicative of Alzheimer's. We had a family conference call. He couldn't get the words out to tell us. All he said was "it's that, it's what we thought." He was crying. We were crying. Though he had shown signs of cognitive decline, there was a weight to the official diagnosis that took my breath away. It had confirmed the inevitable, and now we were faced with the gravity and reality of what was to come.

The problem was that we had *no idea* what was going to come. One of the most challenging aspects of my dad's diagnosis was the unknown. If your loved one has recently been diagnosed with a long-term, degenerative illness, you know exactly what I mean. You are a ball of emotions. Scared, stressed, sad, angry—the whole emotional shebang.

When a loved one is diagnosed with a chronic or progressive illness, it can be emotionally and logistically challenging for the entire family. Conditions like dementia, Parkinson's disease, heart disease, and others may gradually limit a loved one's ability to live independently and care for themselves. As difficult as this is, planning ahead can help ease the transition and reduce stress when the time comes. In retrospect, there was no juncture for our family where we looked back on our experience and said, "Wow, we planned that too early." We made plans for our dad's sixtieth birthday a year in advance, knowing that he likely would not be around for his next big birthday. We made a schedule of visits and caregivers on a month-to-month basis. We looked at home health care options and adult day care even while he was comfortable to be at home. Some of these steps took months to materialize, but by starting early we were able to involve our dad in his future planning while he had more of his mind. As his disease progressed, he was not able to articulate his needs or wants in the same way.

So, if you're reading this, take a deep breath. Yes, the diagnosis likely is awful, but you can take some control over the situation by planning ahead. It will make things a lot easier when stuff gets real. This chapter has got you covered on how to prep for your loved one's health issues. [For a quick reference guide, see our long-term planning checklist in Appendix 1.]

Step 1: Be a part of the conversation

Each situation is different. Were you there when your loved one was diagnosed? Did you get a dreaded phone call like I did? Maybe your mom just casually dropped the news at a family dinner and you were completely shook, or perhaps you're a little estranged from your loved ones and you heard through the grapevine. No matter how tough it is to hear, it will bring about a lot of feelings. Those feelings are unlikely to subside anytime soon, so you need to process them and distract yourself with planning.

However you first found out about your loved one or loved one's illness, it will take some time to process. It is a lot to take in. One of the first steps is to have open and honest conversations with your loved one about their diagnosis, limitations, and wishes for the future. Although you may not agree with some of their preferences and expectations, the sooner you have an open conversation, the sooner you can begin to process how things may shake out. It's important to set realistic expectations, and that starts with knowing what they expect and what you may be capable of doing to support them. Once you understand their preferences, you can plan accordingly.

You'll have to talk a lot in order to understand your loved one's situation. The amount of information that goes into understanding a long-term health condition is *dense*. It is like all those high school classes you wanted to forget about combined into one: you're about to get into the weeds of clinical care needs, indicators of health, home safety issues, and how to pay for all of it. So strap in!

When having initial conversations with your loved one about their diagnosis, stay human. Don't bounce in and start firing off questions like it's a life insurance application. Be empathetic and take it slow. Your loved one is likely processing a lot, as are other members of your family.

Here is a list of key topics to hit on:

- Treatment options and managing medications
- Daily living abilities and needs
- Safety at home
- Future housing and care arrangements
- Financial and legal planning
- Emotional support and counseling

It's understandable if your loved one is reluctant to talk about these topics. Be patient and empathetic, and focus the conversation on how planning ahead will allow them to maintain the highest quality of life possible. They may need time to process the situation. You can try again later, seek support from other family members, or ask their doctor for help to broach sensitive subjects.

Here are two different approaches you can try.

The first is what we will call "The emotional approach." This tactic leads with an emotional connection and an acknowledgment of the challenges of the situation. The use of this style will depend on your own personality and your family dynamics. If you are not a "feel-y" person, this might not be your vibe. However, if feeling heard and seen is important to you and your loved one, this style of communication may be beneficial. Here are some specifics.

- Start with Empathy: begin the conversation by expressing empathy and understanding. Let your loved one know that you care about them and want to support them through this challenging time.
- Keep It Informal: converse in a relaxed manner. Choose a comfortable setting where you both feel at ease, whether it's over a cup of coffee or during a walk in the park or just at home.
- Be Honest and Open: express your concerns and feelings. Let your loved one know why you want to discuss their long-term illness.
- Ask Open-ended Questions: encourage your loved one to share thoughts and feelings. Listen actively and validate their experiences without judgment.
- Offer Support: any kind of support or assistance in any way you can. Let your loved one know that you're there for them and willing to help with practical tasks, emotional support, or just being a listening ear.
- Provide Information: this may concern the illness or available resources. Offer to research treatment options, support groups, or community services together.

- Respect Their Wishes: let your loved one take the lead in making decisions about their care and treatment, and support them in whatever choices they make.
- Follow Up: check in regularly with your loved one on how they're doing and see if there's anything you can do to support them. Keep the lines of communication open and continue to be there for them throughout their illness journey.

The second approach is what we will call "The practical approach." This one is more business-like focused. It may resonate if you and your loved one are do-ers. If you are natural problem solver or want answers to questions, this style of communication may be for you. Here are some specifics.

- Do Your Research: start by educating yourself about your loved one's illness. Use reliable online resources, medical websites, and support forums to learn more about the condition and available treatment options.
- Determine the Format: if you aren't a big talker with your loved one, consider using technology to facilitate the conversation. Consider scheduling a video call if you're unable to meet in person, or use messaging apps to communicate some information you have found.
- Share Resources: share relevant articles, videos, or podcasts with your loved one to help them better understand their illness and what to expect. Encourage them to explore online support groups or forums where they can connect with others facing similar challenges.
- Offer Practical Assistance: offer practical assistance using planners, digital tools, and apps. For example, you could help your loved one set up medication reminders on their smartphone or download fitness and nutrition apps to track their health goals.

- Seek Professional Guidance: encourage your loved one to seek professional guidance from healthcare providers or counselors. Help them schedule appointments, research specialists, or access telemedicine services for virtual consultations.
- Foster Collaboration: encourage your loved one and their healthcare team to work together. Encourage your loved one to ask questions, keep track of their symptoms, and actively participate in their treatment plan.
- Provide Emotional Support: offer emotional support that feels comfortable to you. Send encouraging messages, share uplifting memes or GIFs, or schedule virtual movie nights or game sessions to lift their spirits.
- Respect Their Privacy: your loved one's privacy and boundaries are important. Ensure that they feel comfortable with the level of communication and support you're providing online.

Which approach is for you? Think of it this way: If you prefer to talk first and then make a plan, leading with empathy might be the better fit. If you prefer to plan and then process emotions, the practical approach may be your way to go. Perhaps you will need a little of both.

Keep in mind that whatever initial approach you take, these conversations can feel awkward, at best, and emotionally scarring, at worst. It is especially difficult when the news is fresh for you and your family. But saying something (nice) can be better than saying nothing.

Beyond these initial conversations, the best advice I can give is to show up. Showing up in some capacity can set the tone for showing that you are there to help. Being present allows an ongoing conversation and points at which to touch base both physically and emotionally with your loved one.

Step 2: Healthcare 101

If you have established your right to be involved in your loved one's care (or, as the Beastie Boys would say, you've fought for your right to join the party), it is time to get organized. Organization is personal. Some like to Marie Kondo things; others (like me) prefer organized chaos, much to my husband's chagrin. When it comes to healthcare needs, figure out a system that will work for you, because you are about to try to fit a new full-time job into your existing life.

Most long-term illnesses will involve not just one clinician but a team of clinicians who are supporting different aspects of care: Think of a brain doctor, heart doctor, primary care doctor, lung doctor, occupational therapist, physical therapist, social worker, psychiatrist, and the list goes on. Each provider can actually have something unique to offer in supporting your loved one, but sometimes the distinctions between their services may not be clear. In many cases, a care manager may be available, and this person can serve as a liaison to you and your family and help make recommendations for other providers. Later, we will talk more about navigating the healthcare system. For now, let's focus on staying organized. Here are some steps to consider:

- Get a sturdy file folder or binder to keep important medical paperwork in one place.
- Set up digital folders on your laptop or cloud storage for scans of health docs. Name folders by category like "insurance" and "prescriptions".
- Sign your loved one up for the patient portal through their clinic. This gives you access to test results, appointment records, messaging doctors.
- Create a shared calendar to track doctor visits, prescriptions, medical tasks. Color code appointments or use symbols to differentiate types.

- Request copies of any medical records from specialty doctors to keep on hand. Scan them into your digital filing system.
- Make medication lists with dosages, prescribing doctors, pharmacy info; update anytime there are changes.
- Set medication reminders or alerts on your phone to prompt refills ahead of time.
- Find a pill organizer box to simplify their daily medicine routine if needed.
- Look into apps or websites that help manage conditions, refills, records, costs. Test some out to see if useful.
- Consider a personal health record service that consolidates all medical data in one account.
- Schedule regular check-ins to go over any health or medication questions with your loved one.
- Create a contact list of their care team—who is their main doctor, also known as their primary care provider (PCP), specialists, pharmacist, home health, therapist, etc.

Step 3: Assessing Your Loved One's Non-Medical Needs

Talking with your loved one is critical, but pretty quickly they may become an unreliable narrator. Losing independence sucks and can make a diagnosis even worse. So your loved one may be reluctant to or frankly incapable of keeping you in the loop. You may think that no news is good news, but that would be or could be patently false.

My friend Anna's mom is a perfect example. She hadn't talked to her mom in a few days and was going about her day. Suddenly, she had three missed calls and four voicemails from her mom (yes, that can happen if someone calls too many times and sends themselves to voicemail). Anna called back, expecting her mom to answer and apologize for butt-dialing. Instead, her mom answered while shouting to a voice in the background that Anna didn't recognize. It was pretty terrifying, Anna told me. It sent sheer panic through her body. Anna's brother tracked down their mom (thanks to the Find My Friends app) and found her at a coffee shop close to home; a stranger nearby had stayed with her because she seemed lost. The takeaway: things can be fine one day and not the next, especially if your loved one's diagnosis deals with cognitive decline, so assess their needs and don't take their word for it.

How do you assess their needs? It is essential to keep tabs on changes in your loved one's health, daily activities, safety at home, moods, social life—basically the whole enchilada. Develop some systems to monitor their well-being regularly. Are they struggling with stuff they used to handle no prob? Time to adjust your support strategies. As your loved one's illness progresses, their needs will change. Ongoing assessment allows you to adapt accordingly.

Here are some general areas to monitor:

- Health: track doctor's appointments, medications, symptoms. Notice cognitive, physical, or mood changes.
- Activities of Daily Living: assess if they need help with bathing, dressing, cooking, housework, transportation, etc.
- Home Safety and Accessibility: look for fall risks like rugs or clutter. Install grab bars, rails, ramps, or other accommodations.
- Social and Community Engagement: encourage them to stay active and social for mental stimulation.

Step 3: Evaluating Living Arrangements

As your loved one declines, check if they can still live independently or require assisted living or nursing home care. Maybe they need to move in with family. Yes, it feels awkward and heavy, but assessing their home status helps you make sure they're safe and taken care of.

The evaluation is exactly what it sounds like: a physical evaluation of the space they are living in to see if that space works for them both currently and as they adapt to the condition they are coping with. The logistics will depend on where you live and where your loved one lives, and even if you end up living together, but initially, here is how it may unfold:

- Do a Walkthrough: schedule a home visit and give yourself at least an hour. Bring that geriatric care manager you found on Yelp along for expert advice. Scope the scene—any potential fall hazards like messy floors or stairs without railings. Check the kitchen for cooking safety and fire hazards. Peep the bathroom setup, too.
- Spy on Their Daily Routine: play secret agent and observe your loved one doing daily activities. How's their mobility, bathing, grooming, dressing, and food prep looking? Note any struggles so you can work on solutions.
- Do a Wellness Check: talk to them about their health. New symptoms? Cognition or mood changes? Pain? Write it all down to share with their doctor.
- Evaluate Their Lifestyle: see how socially active they are. Can they drive safely? How's their community mobility for shopping, place of worship, senior center? Maybe more family visits or Uber rides could help.
- Make a Game Plan: write up your assessment findings for the family. Recommend ideas like home modifications, equipment, or services to help them live their best life. Set a reminder to reassess again soon! Level up those caregiving skills.

This evaluation can be critical. Though many families desperately want to keep their loved one living independently as long as possible, it can be super unsafe, both for the person who is sick and for anyone else living in the home. For more details, see Appendix "Assessing a Loved One's Home Health Needs: Action Plan."

Step 4: Legal and Financial Stuff

Is your head spinning at the thought of legal stuff and financial planning? We are groomed to find these things just *so* adult. I remember making a will when my first son was born and thinking, "why do I need a will? It sounds brutally morbid." But here I am, still kicking despite having a legal document that states my wishes should anything happen. Crossing into lawyer land is intimidating. Most of the time, we don't do it unless a big life change is occurring, often not one that we are prepared to handle. If you think about the times when lawyers get involved in life, it's mainly for major life events: home, job, marriage, divorce, kids, finances, and death. Lots of exciting and intimidating events.

Working with a lawyer to help support your loved one has the double whammy of being intimidating and slightly depressing. You and your loved one will have to face head-on some of life's more challenging questions: What are your wishes for end-of-life care? Who in the family has the legal power to make health decisions once your loved one is no longer able to? How will things be paid for and what happens if the money runs out? It sucks to think about, but it is much better to do so before you are emotionally drained and faced with a decision you have not planned for or talked to your loved one about.

Specifically, it is important to consult with an elder law attorney to put proper legal and financial plans in place, such as the following:

• Wills and estate planning
• Medical powers of attorney

- Financial powers of attorney
- Living wills and advanced directives
- Long-term care insurance claims
- Managing bills and assets

Later, we will get deeper into what these things mean and how to approach them. For planning purposes, here is what you need to know. Figure these things out and have these directives in place, allowing your loved one to express their wishes and make things easier for the family later on. Want to know what would suck? Being at the end of life and not knowing if your loved one wishes to be on life support. Or finding the right healthcare facility for your mom, but not being able to have her moved because you don't have the power of attorney. Or how about this one: fighting with your siblings over who has to make a decision about your loved one's healthcare treatment? It can be brutal, but these things are common. I've spoken with countless people of all ages who say they wish they had figured things out amongst themselves and with their sick family member *before* they were in a crappy situation.

Here is a step-by-step approach to begin your planning:

- Do Your Research: don't just Google any old lawyer. Ask your loved one's doctor or hospital for referrals. Check reviews on Yelp or lawyers.com or ask for referrals. Make sure they specialize in elder law.
- Book a Consult: schedule a meeting to discuss your loved one's situation. Explain their illness, limitations, and needs. The lawyer can advise on options. Bring any documents you already have.
- Get Their Affairs in Order: the lawyer can help draft critical legal docs like wills, advance directives, powers of attorney for medical and financial matters. This ensures your loved one's wishes are followed.

- Understand the Money: review your loved one's insurance, savings, and any benefits they qualify for. The lawyer can assist with long-term care insurance claims, managing bills, and protecting assets.
- Stay in the Loop: keep the lawyer updated on your loved one's condition. Reach out with any new questions or changes. Legal needs evolve over time, so keep them in your corner.
- Bring Your Loved One Along: if they're able, having your mom or dad at the meeting is key. This is ultimately about their needs and wants.
- Tag Team It: if siblings are involved, work together and keep each other informed. Multiple perspectives help build the best care plan.

Working with a lawyer may feel uncomfortable at first, but they have the expertise to handle critical issues. With the right guidance, you can ensure your loved one is protected and cared for during this difficult time.

As a note, it can be financially challenging to hire a lawyer or find one to consult with. Increasingly, there are online services available to make these documents and online services that allow for consults with law school graduates for low hourly costs. If that is the option that is available to you, follow the steps outlined above to figure out the wishes of your loved one and family and make them legally binding by using an electronic service to create the documents.

Hand-in-hand with legal planning is financial planning. If you're rolling your eyes because this sounds like another lecture from your WWII Vet Grandpa, I get it. But financial planning is crucial: long-term care is uber-expensive, rarely covered by typical US insurance, and unlikely to be completely covered anywhere else.

Like everything else, planning to take care of a loved one financially requires careful consideration and preparation. We will get into more helpful tips later in the book, but here are the basics:

- Get Familiar with Your Insurance: review your loved one's health insurance, long-term care insurance, and any other policies that could help pay costs. File claims; appeal denials if needed. Call the insurance pros for guidance.

- Dig Into the Loved One's Finances: look at income sources like retirement accounts, social security, and investments. See if any can be converted to cash to pay bills. It's also time to learn about Medicare, Medicaid, and VA benefits.

- Scope Out Assets: make a list of any property, real estate, stocks, or savings accounts the loved one has. Family may need to sell or rent out assets to raise funds eventually.

- Crunch the Numbers: research estimated costs for medications, equipment, in-home care, and nursing facilities. Account for extra expenses like transportation too. Sticker shock is real.

- Visit the Lawyer: hire an elder-law attorney to update important docs like wills, trusts, and powers of attorney. Protect assets and prepare the estate for the future.

- Get Your Files in Order: create physical and digital systems to organize financial paperwork, bills, claims, etc. Tracking everything avoids headaches later.

- Call a Family Meeting: get siblings and relatives together to review the plan and finances. Decide who will make what financial decisions when needed.

- Stay Flexible: check in regularly to reassess the situation as the illness progresses. New needs may require financial adjustments down the road.

It can be overwhelming, but tackling the money stuff head-on can help give you power over the chaos.

We have covered a lot of material in this chapter. The TL;DR is that planning is critical to expectation management. It helps you to impose order in a difficult situation. It helps your loved one to recognize what may be meaningful markers for their care. The best plan is one that is flexible, with lots of checks and balances, and a clear mile marker for when you need to re-evaluate.

For my family, we identified a few re-evaluation indicators for our plan: when Dad couldn't drive, when he couldn't cook or prepare food himself, when he couldn't use the bathroom independently. Kathryn's mom was dealing with ALS and for her family, the indicators were when she was wheelchair bound, when she couldn't use her hands to grasp things, and when she couldn't form words. The markers may look different, but it is helpful to talk about them. A re-evaluation template can also be found in the Appendix.

CHAPTER 4

Balancing

MY FIRST SON WAS BORN SIX MONTHS BEFORE my dad was diagnosed with Alzheimer's, although he was already showing signs of cognitive decline. After the birth, Dad found lots of joy in playing with his grandson, even getting on the floor to demonstrate crawling. He loved playing and grandparenting. In fact, sometimes he seemed more comfortable with a toddler than around adults. There is comfort in the nonjudgmental nature of a child, and an ease and warmth in not requiring full sentences to get your point across. Kids can be an amazing blessing to those in decline.

As I was getting used to parenting. I was also getting used to being a working mom. Striking a balance among parenting, working, and caregiving, as well as supporting my mom and sister who were even more involved with Dad, was always out of reach. It never felt easy or as though I was fully present.

It may sound obvious, but it's worth painting a stark picture of why this balancing act can be so challenging, even for the most amazing caregivers.

Picture this: you are out of the house and on the job eight to six on most days, maybe working from home on Fridays. The work days don't stop just because you have a family crisis going on. You start to miss Zoom because you want to attend a parent's doctor appointments. You miss even more calls because she can no longer drive herself to the doctor and you have to step in. Skipping those meetings for medical appointments makes you anxious about your job performance. Your bosses say they understand, but even a great boss may eventually give you side-eye if you are out too often. You may need to use up all your paid leave to take your mom to treatments. Now your son has a 103-degree fever and needs to go to the doctor. Who is supposed to take him? Still you!

If that sounds familiar, it's because it happens all the time. The constant juggling leaves you drained and feeling like you're failing at everything: work, parenting, and caregiving. It's demoralizing. The search for balance seems futile.

Personally, I tried different ways to make it work. I made a schedule of visits to my parents. I would allocate time to see my dad and give my mom some time to do her errands. I would bring my kids so that he could spend time with them. I made separate visits just to see my mom so that she could vent about her own caregiving role. We could enjoy our time together without a lot of immediate tasks at hand, and I could try to be a bit more supportive of her. I worked a little less. I would drive four hours one morning and four hours back, late at night, for some of these trips. Giving up a random Wednesday or Friday to travel to a few states sometimes felt stressful. Now I wish I had done it more. My retrospective view is that nothing is more valuable than time. And nothing is more finite. Your time with your loved one is fleeting, but in the moment, it feels impossible to make the time.

As I connected with other caregivers, I was reminded of two things. First, not everyone is able to make the time to be a caregiver. That is ok. In fact, it is actually critical to recognize. Ask yourself, how can this be a part of my life? If you work seven to seven in an office five days a week, your time may not be a resource you can offer. So do what you can; maybe sign up for a weekend shift to be with your loved one, or a few evenings a month, or even call on a lunch break. There are other ways to help from afar that are less about time and more about locating or providing resources. You can research support group options, assist in schedule management, provide financial support, or set up transportation options. Be realistic about your time.

In instances where you did not have a good relationship with your loved one before they got sick, finding balance may be even more frustrating. Why are you upending your life for someone who did not support you? That's a tough question to answer (and we won't try), but make sure whatever balance you strike works for *you*. As someone said to me, the caregiver arrangement that you come up with has to work for both parties.

Here's my best suggestion for achieving balance while caregiving. I affectionately call it the CALMER Steps to Balancing Caregiving Responsibility, because the alternative leaves you anything but calm. The steps are: Clarify the 5Ws, Acknowledge the unknown, List your priorities, Make small steps, Encourage support, and Re-evaluate constantly.

Step 1: Clarify the 5Ws

Take stock of what you know, who you know, where you are, when you have time, and how you can take steps about the condition you are facing and your own needs.

- What do you know about the condition you are facing? Consult with your loved one's clinical care team. What is the prognosis?

What is the timeline? Is there a "typical" case? Do you have access to a clinical coordinator? Make these clarifications regular. Never be afraid to ask questions. (More about this in Chapter 3.)

- Who do you know that can be of help to your loved one and yourself? Start by reaching out to friends and family members who may be willing to offer support. Also consider reaching out to organizations to which you have a connection. If your loved one, for example, is a veteran, see if your local Veterans Administration office can be of assistance. Same thing if you belong to a church. Share your caregiving journey, explain your needs, and ask for assistance. Others may be able to provide emotional support, lend a helping hand with caregiving tasks, or simply be there to listen. Make an actual list of people and keep track of what they may be able to offer. This can be either a written list or a Google Doc, where you have each person's name, location, cell, and availability. It might simply be a WhatsApp or text thread of your go-to people. It doesn't need to be rocket science, but you should have the people you can rely on to help in the caregiving process on speed dial, and keep a broader list of individuals who you can tap for specific things. When Stan was caring for his mom, he made a list of roles and responsibilities for each of his six siblings. One brother was responsible for anything within mom's home that needed to be done—repairs, AC/HVAC issues, etc. Another brother took on financial responsibilities and was deputized to share monthly reports with the other siblings. Stan knew it was his two sisters he could count on for day-to-day help; they were who he was constantly texting for assistance. Perhaps most importantly, Stan's best friends picked up his toddlers when he got stuck at appointments. His is one family's example of using one another's skills to shoulder the load. For our family, we relied on a network of cousins to take one-to-two-hour shifts a couple of times a week. This offered short breaks in the day to get an errand done. However you split it, you need to know who can do what, and you need to communicate.

- Where are you physically, and what resources are available there? Do you live close to your loved one? Do you live with three kids and a dog? Maybe you have roommates? There are going to be physical barriers to your ability to be a caregiver, either because you have other responsibilities or because you don't have the resources to do everything you want to do. Perhaps you don't have regular access to a vehicle, or if you do, the vehicle is full of car seats and can't fit your mom's wheelchair in the trunk. If you are not geographically able to be supportive in day-to-day tasks, don't beat yourself up about it. Instead, think about what you can do from where you are, and what other physical supports are close by. In some geographic areas, there are elder- or community-based services that can drive those who are ill to appointments. Look for these in your own neighborhood. In some localities, there will be a greater availability of community services like volunteer organizations, neighborhood groups, and even visiting health agencies that you can rely on. Where your loved one is living can determine what options you have for outside support.

- When can you be there? Connected to the where are you is when can you be there. A long-term illness is going to be an evolving situation. As soon as you think the schedule is down, it may change. It's the same with a kid's routine in those early years: first they nap all the time, then three times a day, then two, then one, and then, all of a sudden, they are constantly awake. The needle is always moving with a loved one needing care. And if you work or have other responsibilities, your time may be fixed. Block on your calendar the windows in which you can consistently make time and take ownership of caregiving responsibilities during those hours. As mentioned, I was not living in the same state as my parents when my dad was diagnosed. That was really hard. I felt guilty. I would not be able to drive him to appointments or give him his morning, midday, and nighttime meds. All I could do was make a schedule of visits, and add some consistency to those visits, so there were clear windows when other caregivers would have my support.

- Finally, how can you go about tackling these challenges? Consider what you are good at and how that applies to caregiving. Are you super organized? An Excel whiz? That may help you stay on top of appointments, medications, and to-dos. Great! Maybe organization is not your strength, but you are emotionally available? Compassionate? Patient and supportive? This, too, can be useful! Or maybe you are physically capable of helping your loved one with mobility issues and similar tasks. Consider your logistic, emotional, and physical strengths and weaknesses as you set boundaries around being a caregiver.

Step 2: Acknowledge the unknown

Even with the best medical team, most long-term illnesses come with unknowns. Many of them. Our dad was given five to fifteen years to live upon diagnosis. That's an insanely broad timeline, and he ultimately lived only three years. Even wide ranges can be wrong.

In my experience, it is critical to recognize that often you will not have clear answers to your most pressing questions, especially around how quickly the illness will progress and what support you will need. Write down your open questions. Revisit them.

There will also be a lot of information voids. It can be hard to know where to turn with your questions. Dr. Google may be your first impulse but, in this case, you will want to get information from the most reliable sources at all times. It is critical that you identify trusted online resources where you can find out more about your loved one's illness. Start with a professional organization or a non-profit that focuses on the disease you're working with. Also look for a hospital or medical facility that puts content on its website. These sources may not answer all of your specific questions, but they can be a helpful place to start.

Do not take medical action based on something you read on the internet. There is a lot of false content online. Sometimes it is obvious, and other times it is not. The last thing your loved one needs is a steady diet exclusively of fish brains because an influencer said that it was a good idea. After researching something online, bring it to your loved one's next appointment. It goes without saying but

Step 3: List your priorities

There are probably an endless number of things you feel you need to do. Having priorities will help you to decide where to go next. Numerous caregivers who are working full-time experience health issues, depression, and reduced productivity. If you're caring for an elderly or unwell family member, you might notice that you're backing out of community activities or are spending less time with close friends and family members. Here are some tips for setting priorities.

- Communicate clearly with your employer about your caregiving responsibilities and discuss any necessary adjustments to your work schedule or workload. This will help set realistic expectations and allow for potential accommodations.
- Establish clear boundaries between your work and caregiving roles. Define your work hours and communicate those boundaries to your employer, your colleagues, and your loved ones.

Avoid multitasking during work hours and dedicate specific time blocks for caregiving tasks.

- Explore flexible work arrangements, such as flex-time, compressed workweeks, or remote work options, if available. Discuss these options with your employer to find a solution that allows you to fulfill your work responsibilities while managing caregiving duties.
- Consider quality of life. Medical advice can sometimes be inconsistent with quality of life. For example, Dad got very sick on his first Alzheimer's medication. It was impacting his ability to move and keep food down. He ultimately made the choice, while still of sound mind, to stop the medication even though it would likely quicken his decline. At a later time, he chose to eat sweets, even though sugar inhibits brain health, simply because he loved them.

For some, the first priority is identifying a support system: who will help with care, cooking, transportation. For others, the first priority is social and emotional help. Still others will first want to deal with work life. Whatever is most important to you, create a daily or weekly schedule that outlines both your work tasks and caregiving responsibilities. Prioritize tasks based on urgency and importance, and allocate specific time blocks for each activity. This will help you stay organized and focused on your responsibilities.

Step 4: Take small steps

Figuring out how to achieve your priorities is the hardest part. Often you are overwhelmed and in new territory. So start small. Identify someone you already know who may be available to help once a week. Start ordering groceries so you don't need to make a daily run.

Ask your local pharmacy for pill packs so you can stay organized. Small things are in your control, even when the big stuff is not.

Small steps are also critical for self-care, which you'll need to practice to better manage your responsibilities and maintain your physical, mental, and emotional well-being. Here are some small steps for self-care:

- Get Some Sleep. Quality sleep is life. We are learning that lack of sleep can contribute to the development of cognitive decline— Yikes! Set a chill bedtime routine so you can wind down. That might mean dimming lights, herbal tea, calming podcasts, or whatever works for you. If nights are when you're on duty and they're interfering with your sleep, talk to family members or professionals about getting night-shift help so you can catch some uninterrupted sleep.
- Step Away. Don't let caregiver duties take over your whole life! Schedule breaks. Leave things with in-home help, family assistance, or temporary professionals. Use that you-time to recharge doing something you love. Think about Rema. She did not want to miss out on her son's soccer games, so she consistently had her neighbor stay with her mom while she attended. She always left an hour earlier than necessary for the games so she could grab a coffee and listen to her favorite podcast before the game began. She would just sit in her car and relax. She needed it. It was her Zen time.
- Stress Less. When anxiety strikes, have quick calm-down routines like breathwork, meditation apps, or yoga flows. Find moments of quiet to reset throughout your insane days.
- Let Emotion In. Being a caregiver is rough and comes with *all* the emotions. Don't bottle them up! Write in a journal, call a friend, join an online support group to vent. It's healthy. A great friend sent me a mindfulness journal where each morning I

would write down something good and bad and look forward to the day. I loved it. Another friend told me she would start each morning writing down something funny her kids did the day before, and it would remind her that even as she was watching her dad ail, she was watching her kids grow.

- Set Boundaries. You can't pour from an empty cup, fam. Set limits to protect your time and well-being. Say "no" more. Ask for help. Don't take on too much. Communicate your needs.
- Do You. Make time for hobbies and activities that are 100 percent for you. Not chores or errands. Read, game, binge Netflix, craft—whatever feeds your soul and recharges you. Feeling isolated is brutal and can lead to declining health for you as a caregiver. Find and sustain your support network who gets your caregiver journey.
- Find a Professional. If you're struggling, there's zero shame in seeking professional counseling help. Having an expert listen and provide tools is healthy. Don't tough it out alone. Jeff had been committed to therapy since he was seventeen, but when he was twenty-four and his dad was diagnosed with Parkinson's disease and began to seriously decline faster than expected, he upped his sessions. The point is, make sure your mental health plan is meeting your changing needs.

Taking care of yourself makes you a stronger and more sustainable caregiver.

Step 5: Build Your Tribe

I know you may not have listed finding support as a top priority, but it can be absolutely critical. Coping with illness is not a short-term deal and being a caregiver can leave you feeling isolated. Having people in your corner who truly get what you're going through is so important. But between taking care of your parent and all your other adulting duties, it's hard to find time to connect. That's why it is critical to get strategic about building your tribe. We already talked about rallying your crew. This is your siblings, cousins, aunts/ uncles, friends, anyone close who can lend a hand. Even if they can't physically help out, they provide love and trusted ears. But there are other forms of support that you may be less comfortable or familiar with.

- Join Support Groups. Look for local support groups or online communities specifically for caregivers. These groups provide a platform for sharing experiences, seeking advice, and finding empathy from others going through similar situations. You can connect with caregivers who understand the challenges you face and offer valuable insights and support.
- Check Out Caregiver Events, Workshops, and Conferences in Your Area. These gatherings often provide opportunities to meet and connect with other caregivers, learn from expert speakers, and gain valuable knowledge and resources. Participating can expand your network and provide a sense of community. Meeting people who have all different reactions and experiences to caretaking can help normalize the emotions that come with caregiving.
- Explore Online Websites, Forums, and Social Media Groups Dedicated to Caregiving. They can offer a wealth of information, support, and opportunities to connect with other caregivers. Engage in discussions, ask questions, and share your experiences to build connections and gain insights from the online caregiving community.
- Ask the Professionals. Consider reaching out to pros who specialize in caregiving, such as social workers, therapists, or counselors. They can provide guidance, emotional support, and strategies

to navigate the challenges of caregiving. They may also be able to connect you with additional resources and support networks.

- Connect with Volunteer Organizations. Research local volunteer groups or community centers that offer support services to caregivers. Connecting with these organizations can not only provide an opportunity to give back but also allow you to connect with fellow caregivers and build a support network within the organization.
- Be a Student. Participate in caregiver training programs or educational workshops offered by healthcare providers, community centers, or organizations. These programs not only provide valuable knowledge and skills but also offer opportunities to connect with other caregivers who are seeking similar education and support. Many organizations offer free trainings for caregivers.

Step 6: Re-evaluate consistently

Again, long-term illness is dynamic. Prognoses can change. Mary's mom was diagnosed with general dementia. For months she was able to hold a full-time job and live on her own, then for months after she would forget how to drive. The whiplash was astounding. You may notice differences in your loved one more quickly than you thought you would. You may also realize that what you thought would work for your family is no longer the case. It's critical to re-evaluate and follow the CALMER steps as things move. You likely have multiple responsibilities to juggle, including caregiving, parenting, work, and other commitments. Re-evaluating how you are coping allows you to assess the balance of these responsibilities and make adjustments as needed to prevent burnout and maintain your own well-being.

Summing Up

It is possible to balance your new role as a caregiver and person. The *CALMER Steps to Balancing Caregiving Responsibility* are an approach I developed based on my own experience and countless conversations with others in similar positions. The steps are listed in the Chapter 4 Appendix. Remember, only you can find the right balance between yourself and your family. And keep in mind that things are more likely to feel like a seesaw than a balance beam. You'll need a lot of introspection and evaluation as the disease changes. Reserve the right to change your mind because, just as a child's needs evolve as they grow, the needs of a family member receiving long-term care change over time, and your needs as a caregiver will change, too.

CHAPTER 5

Effective Communication and Family Dynamics

B Y NATURE, PEOPLE COMMUNICATE IN DIFFER-
ENT ways. They cope in different ways. They have different
capacities—time, skill, empathy. There will likely be one
(maximum two) person in the family who is the primary caregiver.
It becomes an exercise of radical acceptance to trust that they are
doing the best they can, in the only way they know how, to support
the ailing person. It is critical to realize that things will not be equal
among adult children and siblings in the caregiving role, and that
each will act and react to others according to their individual nature.

My friend Rose has a brother who has always been a happy-go-
lucky, rose-colored-glasses sort of guy. He was getting married and
starting his life far away from their parents in Maine. His visits home
were relatively limited. Rose got frank with him. He needed to be
more physically present. After that conversation, he made a change,
kudos to him. Some siblings might have been deeply offended. Rose's

brother just needed to hear it directly before he would take action, not because he didn't care, but because he's the kind of guy who sees what is good, not what is bad. The problems Rose was dealing with weren't his focus until they had to be. This was a pre-existing family dynamic, and it had to be addressed head-on.

Thinking about innate approaches to life, I would call myself a problem solver. I am what we described in Chapter 3 as someone who takes the practical approach. When I encounter a problem, I like to move ASAP to solutions. I thrive by doing. This is not the case for my sister. It's not that she avoids problems or enjoys sitting with them. Rather, she wants to listen and think before reacting and solving. She is more responsive to an empathetically oriented conversation. Our respective strategies mean that in our conversations we need to recognize what each of us is looking for—whether to talk or problem-solve—and react accordingly.

Communication is often dismissed as something we all do. It shouldn't be. It is complicated. It is both an art and a science. There are abundant social science theories dedicated to interpersonal communication. For instance, Attachment Theory, developed by Bowlby and Ainsworth, which explores how early relationships with caregivers influence patterns of communication and behavior in adult relationships (Bowlby, J., 1969, "Attachment and Loss"). So much of who we are and how we interact with others is connected to our bonds with our earliest caregivers—usually our parents. That's what makes communication about and with loved ones exceptional, for better or worse. It's why many of our greatest vulnerabilities come out when we're communicating about our parents as they ail.

Communication cannot make up for bad decisions, but knowing how that decision is reached can significantly change perceptions of motivations, and how people feel about decisions. Think about how many times in daily life you disagree with someone else's choice. Let's say you and your coworker have to make a tough call on a project.

You think you should wait two days before submitting a proposal to your client so that your boss can review it; your coworker wants to send it to the client today. And she submits it. You are dumbfounded. Why would she do that?! You approach your coworker, pissed. She explains that she submitted the proposal because she knew the client looked favorably on first offers and a competitor was lurking with a rival submission. Maybe you still are pissed at your coworker, but her reasoning may make the decision seem tolerable.

What's the point? Communicating about reasons and rationales can be constructive. The same premise applies to nearly every aspect of caregiving. You will inevitably have differing opinions with other members of your family, perhaps even with professionals, about your loved one's care. It's critical to effectively communicate about the why and come to a shared understanding.

Navigating Family Dynamics

Nearly every caretaker I have met has a story about a misunderstanding or frustration among family, friends, or others involved in the care. Caregiving involves adults who are doing their best to balance their own lives while accepting a radical new world for someone they love. Things get stressful. We often take out that stress on those closest to us. Sometimes it is warranted, and sometimes not.

My colleague, Jace, and his sister, Sosie, were dealing with their dad's Parkinson's diagnosis. Said Sosie:

> When our dad was diagnosed with Parkinson's disease last year, my brother and I wanted to ensure we could both help care for him. I work close by as a teacher, so I volunteered to visit dad on my way home from school to prepare dinner. My brother has a busy job and two young kids, so he offered to take dad to

his neurology and physical therapy appointments. This system worked for the first few months, but gradually issues came up. I started feeling overwhelmed, juggling my job, caring for my own family, and making dad's meals daily. I wrongly assumed my brother was checking on dad regularly since he handled medical transportation. Meanwhile, my brother thought I was keeping a closer eye on dad's overall condition since I saw him daily. He didn't realize how much dad was declining cognitively and physically. Dad's needs were increasing. Things were *not* working. We finally had a come-to moment and realized neither of us had the full picture. Now we have a shared calendar to track dad's appointments and needs. We split up some of the care tasks more evenly and check in at least weekly about additional support we may need from other family or professionals.

When I asked Sosie about ways in which communication helped or hindered her relationship with Jace, she said "being intentional about communication is key, especially when we're balancing busy work lives. It's a continual process as dad's condition progresses."

Families are complicated in the best of times. Communication in families can become especially complicated in caregiving situations. Family dynamics can change. An ailing person can shift roles within the family. The person assuming the caregiving role may have to make decisions and take on responsibilities that were previously held by other family members. This shift in power dynamics can create tension as family members adjust to their new roles. Each family member will have different expectations and values when it comes to caregiving. Differences in beliefs about the appropriate level of care, the allocation of resources, or even the importance of the caregiving role itself can lead to conflicts and misunderstandings.

Family dynamics, of course, are often shaped by past experiences and unresolved conflicts. These issues can resurface or become magnified during the caregiving process, adding an additional layer of complexity. If, for instance, caregiving places a significant burden on one or a few family members, they may burnout or feel resentful, or both unequal distribution of caregiving responsibilities can strain relationships.

Similar to Jace and Sosie's experience, was a story my friend Candace told me about her family: Our mom was diagnosed with renal disease two years ago and it was a shock. Then she began showing signs of dementia last year, and we knew caregiving would be even more challenging. Me and my sisters each have different life circumstances. Sarah works full time and has two young children. Emily is a stay-at-home mom with a flexible schedule. I live across the country in California, working as an art teacher and trying to finish my studio series. We always bickered as kids because we are *so* different. As adults, it was better—we each did our own thing—but it's pretty obvious that we are still different in what we want in life and how we run our day-to-day. Naturally, tensions started rising over our mom's care. Emily resented always being the one relied on to take mom to dialysis and doctor visits, just because she had the most flexible schedule. I could only visit so often from California, but felt guilty not being around more. Sarah was juggling work and raising kids, leaving her barely any bandwidth to assist, but also somewhat pissed at how Emily was handling things. Our group text arguments about who was doing what for mom got heated. It took a family counseling session for us all to air our grievances and frustrations productively. We have done our best to resolve the communication challenges, but tensions can still get high. We have an app where we document mom's daily needs. We each are commitment to checking it every day. We have a text strategy where we message "SOS" if the alert is critical and extra help is needed. We try to divide tasks fairly based on availability. If someone can't take on something, we cover for each. I think the judgement and resentment are still there but we hide it better. It's an ongoing balancing act. I wouldn't say things resolved, but they came to a stable place for now. With each change in mom's care, I would say we need to re-balance how we talk to each other and who does what. It's not static.

Adding to the immense amount of stress that caregiving brings are financial considerations, such as managing medical expenses, making housing modifications, or paying for professional care services. Disagreements over how to allocate financial resources can lead to conflict within the family. Questions that might easily be resolved in normal times can potentially lead to heightened emotions and disputes in a caregiving environment.

Because every family is different, the ways in which conflict arises under the stress of caregiving will be different. In almost every situation, however, insufficient or ineffective communication will exacerbate tensions and create new ones, while open and honest communication will tend to help you address issues and work together as a cohesive caregiving team. Here are some tips for communicating amid complicated family dynamics:

- Foster Openness and Honesty among Family Members. Emphasize the importance of respectful communication. Create a safe space where everyone feels comfortable expressing their thoughts and concerns. Rose and her brother are the perfect example here. Had Rose not expressed the need for her brother to visit more, she would have resented him to this day. A simple act of honesty saved a future relationship.
- ! Practice Active Listening. All family members involved in the conversation should be heard. Pay attention to their perspectives,

emotions, and underlying concerns. Just because something is not emotionally taxing for you doesn't mean that it's not that way for others. Validate their feelings and strive to understand their point of view, even if you disagree. I watched this first hand. My mom and sister were both caregivers for my dad. Their emotional experiences were very different. It took a lot of open communication, and a lot of listening both ways, to get through the caregiving process together.

- Choose the Right Timing and Setting. Choose a neutral and private location that allows for focused discussions. Avoid sensitive topics during times of high stress or when emotions are running high. In our family, this meant we always had important conversations at home, whether in person or on the phone. Even if an incident occurred in a public place, we would do our best to limit the discussion and processing of it until we were in a safe and comfortable place. I still vividly recall Dad losing it at a restaurant and wandering into a space he wasn't supposed to be in, then refusing to leave. The rest of us differed in what we thought should be done—force him to leave, or take a more laissez-faire approach. We did our best to align in the moment through nonverbal communication and saved the talk for later when the emotional stakes would be lower.

- Use "I" Statements. When expressing your thoughts or concerns, speak for yourself to avoid sounding accusatory or confrontational. Say "I feel . . ." or "I am concerned about . . ." instead of making sweeping statements, speaking for others, or attacking others. We all say the wrong things at some point in our caregiving experiences. If we all followed this rule, we'd do so less frequently. It is critical to acknowledge that we only really know our own feelings, and that making generalizations can cause others to shut down.

- Set Boundaries and Enforce Them. What is acceptable behavior and communication within the family? It's best to discuss this openly and respectfully, and to be consistent in enforcing the rules. Boundaries help maintain respectful interactions and healthy dynamics. We generally would not contact each other when someone was on break—say, Mom was out to dinner with friends while we were with Dad—unless it was a true emergency. Respecting this boundary allowed the person who was "off" to know that if we did, in fact, reach out, it was truly a last resort.

- Focus on Common Goals and Shared Interests. Identifying them among family members will highlight areas of agreement. Emphasize the importance of working together to meet the needs and well-being of the loved one receiving care. Our common goal was keeping Dad safe. My sister felt strongly that he needed to be supervised 24/7 at home. Our mom felt that wasn't realistic (and it wasn't). Even though we disagreed, understanding that we had the same goal was helpful in us discussing how to best supervise him realistically.

- Practice Empathy and Understanding. Recognize that everyone's experiences and emotions are valid, even if they differ from your own. It can help to try to understand the underlying concerns and motivations behind family members' actions or reactions. For instance, the loss that you and your loved one are experiencing will be different. Caregiving alongside an able parent forced us to recognize the different types of loss, and the complicated loss that our mom was experiencing and which was affecting her day-to-day.

- Manage Conflict Constructively. Encourage open dialogue, active listening, and problem-solving, rather than resorting to blame or defensiveness. Use "we" language to emphasize the shared goal of finding a resolution. Things like "we" have to work through this together. Be prepared for more than one conversation. In our family, we didn't always get it right on the first try. The important thing was to come back the next time and be more constructive. We always were able to come to a solution, even if it took a few rounds.

- Consider Professional Support. If family dynamics remain highly challenging, try a family therapist or counselor who specializes in working with families facing complex dynamics. A professional can provide guidance, facilitate productive discussions, and help the family develop healthier communication patterns. Prior to my dad's diagnosis, my sister was most comfortable with her own emotional needs. She encouraged everyone to seek their own form of therapy.

Communicating with Your Loved One

Before becoming a caregiver, one thing I couldn't fathom was how hard it would become to communicate with my dad. He was always kind, caring, calm, although a man of few words. It was pretty easy to talk to him. Early in his condition, he would do his best to communicate with his family and friends. He was still able to follow a conversation, although his vocal contributions were limited. Later on, he might chime in with a thought, something that had taken him a few minutes to pull together. By then, the conversation had moved on. You could see the glee on his face when he got the words out, and then the disappointment when he realized by looking at others that his words had not met the moment. Eventually, it became challenging for him to even follow extended conversations with multiple others, so he adopted nonverbal behaviors, shaking his head, or a brief smile. One-on-one, he could still get many thoughts across. He would gesture, point, or laugh. When he met my second child, just six months before he died, he stated quite loudly that his new grandson looked like my brother had as a baby. The words flowed effortlessly. Then he was back to nodding and smiling. Eventually, those nonverbal cues started to make less sense. His entire temperament changed with his disease. He would become irate for no reason. He would fixate on the smallest things and repeat himself over and over again when he did have words. Communicating with your loved one as they decline is challenging. It is time-consuming and emotionally taxing. My friend Dana told me about her experience communicating with her mother:

Caring for my mom has been the hardest thing I've ever done. When she was diagnosed with dementia last year, I stepped up right away to be her primary caregiver. I manage her medical appointments, make her meals, help her with daily tasks—anything she needs. But her dementia has completely changed her personality. She regularly says critical, hurtful things to me that she never would have said before. I know it's the illness, but her words still pierce me. Like when I cook her favorite dinner after a long day and she yells that it's bland and disgusting. Or when I help her get ready for bed and she snaps that I'm clumsy and useless.

In the moment, I have to take deep breaths and remind myself it's not my real mom saying these things. But when you're constantly criticized by the person you're trying to care for, it's crushing. I end up feeling worthless and burnt out. I don't want to give up on her. She's still my mother and I know she'd take care of me if the roles were reversed. But setting boundaries is difficult when her put-downs come unpredictably.

I asked Dana how she was coping with this. "I'm learning I have to prioritize my mental health, too," she said. "Now I ask a family member or friend to join some of the time when I visit, so I'm not the sole target of her dementia-fueled criticism. I also limit visits to her best time of day when she seems more cheerful whenever I can, but sometimes that is just not practical.

It's an imperfect solution and my feelings still get hurt regularly. But caring for someone with dementia means protecting yourself, too. I'm trying to remember my worth has nothing to do with her illness-driven words. Some days that's easier said than done."

Below are ten suggestions for communicating with someone who is experiencing cognitive decline. Most are also useful when caring for anyone who is dealing with long-term illness and exhibiting a change in temperament or other repercussions from their illness:

- Use Simple Language. Speak clearly and use straightforward sentences. Avoid using complex words or phrases that might confuse the person. Dad seemed to consistently recognize the word "misunderstanding," so we would try to use that term in explaining something.

- Maintain Eye Contact. Establishing eye contact conveys your attention and interest. This helps in making the person feel more secure and valued during the conversation.

- Be Patient. People with dementia or people in pain or on medication may take longer to understand and respond. Wait patiently for their reply without rushing them, and avoid interrupting or finishing their sentences. Suggesting a term or phrase may be beneficial, but avoid rushing to fill their void.

- Use Nonverbal Cues. Body language, facial expressions, and tone of voice can all convey meaning more effectively sometimes than words alone. Use positive nonverbal cues to support your speech. This will not work in all situations—sometimes those experiencing cognitive decline will lose the ability to recognize cues. In these instances, it may help to guide them with soft physical touch.

- Avoid Correcting or Arguing. If the person makes mistakes or remembers things incorrectly, let it pass. Arguing can cause distress. It's often more beneficial to enter their reality and engage with them from their perspective. Dad would often say that he was alone for hours. In fact, he simply couldn't find one of us in the house. There was no value in confronting this.

- Focus on Feelings, Not Facts. Pay attention to the emotions behind what the person is saying. Even if their words are confused, they can still express how they feel. Acknowledge and validate these feelings.

- Use Names. To avoid confusion, use proper names instead of pronouns such as "he" or "she" when talking about others. Similarly, identify yourself and others directly by name.

- Limit Distractions. Reduce background noise to make it easier for the person with dementia to focus on the conversation. Dad would like to keep the TV on or music playing from his phone, which perhaps helped with loneliness, but it also made conversations impossible.

- Engage in Activities. Shared activities can facilitate communication. Engage in simple, enjoyable tasks together like looking through photo albums, gardening, or listening to music. My sister and Dad would watch football together (despite it probably being low on her interest list), but it allowed dad to be "the leader" of the conversation because he knew more about the sport and could pull some insane memories out of nowhere.

- Use Reminiscence. Talking about past experiences can be comforting and easier for people with dementia. Their long-term memory often remains stronger than short-term memory. It can be helpful to focus on particularly unique memories. Our family had taken an extensive white water rafting trip a decade ago. Dad loved to talk about it.

Communicating beyond the Family

Talking to friends about what you're going through as a caregiver is important. You'll receive support and understanding, and it will help to maintain your own well-being. At the same time, it can be emotionally taxing to repeat yourself and your experience over and over. If it's helpful to you, write it out, almost like a script. It may take some of the spontaneity out of your presentation, but it can conserve your emotional energy.

When you are up for it, here are some strategies to effectively communicate with friends:

- Choose the Right Time and Place. Remember that, you have the right to say "let's talk about that at a different time." Choose a comfortable and private setting to have an open conversation, and pick a time when you can dedicate your full attention to the discussion without distractions.
- Be Open and Honest. Share your thoughts and feelings with your friends. Let them know about your challenges and emotions, and the impact caregiving is having on your life. Avoid minimizing or downplaying your experiences. As a society, we are not honest when people ask, "how are you?" We are expected to say "good, and you?" But it's okay to be frank in conversations, however surprising it may be to others. You have a right to be direct with people, if that feels comfortable for you.
- Educate Them about Caregiving. Your friends may not be familiar with what it requires. Provide them with some background information about your loved one's condition, the tasks involved in caregiving, and the impact it has on your life. This can help them better understand your situation and empathize with your experiences. Prepare for questions that seem out of touch, mundane, or that piss you off. It will happen.

- Be Specific about Your Needs. Clearly communicate what kind of support or help you would appreciate from your friends. It could be you need practical assistance with specific tasks, or emotional support, or simply someone to listen without judgment. Let them know what they can do to be there for you in a meaningful way.
- Practice Active Listening. Allow your friends to share their thoughts and feelings in response to your experiences. When my mom's siblings told her they were concerned about her wellbeing, it took some time, but she listened and started taking more breaks. Give friends your full attention, ask follow-up questions, and validate their responses. This can deepen your connection and foster a two-way supportive relationship.
- Share Updates and Progress. Keep friends informed about your caregiving journey, including any updates or progress you experience. Sharing milestones, challenges, and positive moments can help them feel connected and involved in your life as a caregiver.
- Set Boundaries. While it's important to share your experiences, also establish boundaries if there are certain aspects you prefer to keep private. Communicate your comfort levels and let your friends know what topics or details are off-limits for discussion. Remember that you are in control of the conversation.
- Seek Support Groups or Online Communities. Encourage your friends to join you in caregiver support groups or online communities. This can provide them with insights into your experiences and allow them to connect with other caregivers. It can also help them gain a broader understanding of caregiving and find ways to offer support. My mom found some solace in a spousal support group, although the older age of the other attendees meant that she did not always have her needs met. My sister, on the other hand, was so connected to her support group, she has now become a peer leader.

- Be Patient with Responses. At first, friends may not fully comprehend the complexities of caregiving. Give them time to process the information and adjust their understanding. Be patient if they struggle to offer the support you need, but also be open to having ongoing conversations to help them better understand your situation.
- Express Gratitude. Show appreciation for your friends' willingness to listen and support you, and for their efforts, big or small, in being there for you during your caregiving journey.

These are just the basics for communicating about caregiving. You may find it easier to keep others updated through a social media page, a WhatsApp group, or other forms of outbound communication. You may find that you actually don't have the energy to communicate much about your experience and that is also ok. Communication is a means to elicit support or understanding, but it is not a requirement.

Summing It Up

Communication can be the difference between an effective care team able to support your loved one and each other, and a family meltdown as a result of caregiving. Some families cannot get over their differences to make unified decisions. Others do not survive the caregiving experience as an intact unit. This compounds the losses associated with an ailing loved one. Prioritizing communication approaches can help to avoid this worst-case scenario.

CHAPTER 6

Healthcare Management and Advocacy

I HAD SOME FAMILIARITY WITH THE MEDICAL SYSTEM because of my educational background. Nothing prepares you for having to navigate it on behalf of someone else. Most medical systems, including those of the United States, are fragmented, poorly incentivized, and incredibly complex. When dealing with a complicated medical issue that will not be treated by one physician, be prepared for an uphill battle.

We were connected with a patient navigator who served as a point person to the neurologist managing my dad's Alzheimer's care. We would call her when medication was not working or we noticed changes in Dad's progression. We independently needed to find a psychiatrist to deal with the depression that came from his knowing that he was declining. And he still had to see his regular cardiologist and primary care physician. It was easy to lose count of the medical appointments, medications, and emergency room visits that were required to support Dad's care.

Millennials and the Healthcare System

Younger adults have distinct ways of engaging with the medical system, and they don't exactly jive with supporting someone else's care. Millennials utilize healthcare services in ways that reflect their comfort with technology and preference for convenience. They are more likely to seek information and initial diagnoses online, often using reputable health websites and telehealth services to consult doctors virtually. One study found that 67.2 percent of millennials read online reviews before selecting a physician.[7] This makes it less likely for younger adults to have visited a healthcare facility for their own health compared to older adults. Other research says that millennials utilize healthcare services less than older generations and are more likely to rely on urgent care or emergency room.[8] At the same time, millennials who do see a primary care doctor for, say, an annual check-up report higher satisfaction rates with their provider than older generations.[9]

Additionally, millennials are more likely to switch healthcare providers if they feel their needs are not being met, prioritizing providers who offer online appointment scheduling, electronic health records, and email or messaging communication. Sometimes younger adults will even turn to social media to find recommendations for healthcare providers and share experiences with providers, creating crowd-sourced feedback on care.

While these behaviors may make sense for your own health, they don't necessarily fit when dealing with someone else's care. You may have limited options when it comes to finding a local provider that can address your loved one's particular illness. Within the geographic area our family lived in, there were two primary medical facilities, each with several doctors who specialized in Alzheimer's care and coordination. In some areas, there may be fewer options. So while it may be beneficial to crowd-source recommendations, you may need to work with providers available to you unless you are willing to travel and a special provider elsewhere has availability and is covered by your insurance.

Young adults are also less likely to be comfortable with the medical system simply because they tend to be healthier and access it less frequently. All of this means that millennials may be interacting with a super-complicated, in-person medical system for the first time on behalf of their loved one. The learning curve may be steep.

Healthcare Navigation and Advocacy

Here are some notes that may be helpful in navigating the US healthcare system.

Health Insurance. Start with some basic questions. Does your loved one have health insurance? If so, great! That means some of your loved one's medical expenses will be covered. How much will be covered depends on the type of health insurance and the parameters of the particular insurance plan. The private health insurance typically provided by an employer, or bought in a private insurance market, is offered by large insurance companies such as UnitedHealthcare, Aetna, and Cigna. Each of these providers has different types of health plans, each requiring different amounts of out-of-pocket spending (deductibles) before the health insurance covers services. It is critical to understand the parameters of your loved one's health insurance as you get involved in this space. Make a call to whomever is offering the plan and ask for an explanation of benefits. Ask whatever questions you can think of until you get the clarity on what is covered and what you will pay for. There will be in-network and out-of-network expenses for both health plans. In-network expenses will cost you less but also tend to provide less access to specialty doctors. In addition to deductibles, you will learn about co-pays and premiums. If your loved one is over sixty-five, they qualify for Medicare, which is provided by the US government and offers hospital coverage (at a minimum). Many adults over sixty-five also have supplemental insurance coverage. Depending on income level or disability status, your loved one may also have Medicaid, which is for individuals who are below a particular income threshold. All of this will take time to investigate.

Identify and Work with a Care Team. Where is the best place for your loved one to get care? Maybe they already have a doctor who is supporting them in their diagnosis. Sometimes it is a general medicine doctor who has flagged your loved one's symptoms and referred them to a specialist. If you need to find a care team, check out the websites of your local hospital or contact your insurance provider to identify in-network specialists who can address your loved one's needs. Again, start in your insurance network to avoid paying a lot more. Even when you find a doctor, getting an appointment can take weeks or even months, especially with specialists.

Rely on Patient Navigators. Often, many insurance companies and providers will connect you with a patient navigator for complex, long-term conditions. This person will serve as your main point of contact to address the multiple complex needs of your loved one. It can be helpful to have a patient navigator, and you may want to seek one out regardless. Keep them informed of what's going on and rely on their recommendations when you can.

Communicate with Providers. Ask yourself another question: How can you get up to speed to best communicate with your provider? Medical terms and jargon are hard to understand, making it difficult to know what treatments and procedures your loved one needs. This is a space that you can work on independently. Before appointments or discussions with healthcare providers, make a list of questions, concerns, and important information you want to discuss. If you have your provider's email address, you can send them in advance. You are your loved one's advocate, so anything you have noticed that is confusing or seems out of the ordinary is fair game to discuss. It can be helpful to provide specific examples to help healthcare providers understand the situation better. Take notes during conversations to help you remember important details, and leverage technology—patient portals, email, or telehealth platforms—for better communication with healthcare providers. More on digital tools in Chapter 7.

Organize the Finances. The paperwork involved in patient care can be another big hurdle. When visiting a doctor or hospital, you are often given a stack of forms to fill out, asking for detailed health and insurance information. After your visit, the billing process is complex. Your loved one might receive multiple bills from different providers for one visit, and the charges can be confusing. You could get a bill from the hospital, another from the doctor, and another from the lab that did your blood tests, each with different amounts you owe. All billing information should be shared with your loved one's insurance provider and organized in a physical folder or electronically so you can keep track of expenses.

Keep Medical Records and Medication Information. Organizing your loved one's medical information can help you keep track of important details, facilitate communication with healthcare providers, and ensure comprehensive care. You may want to set up a dedicated physical binder or folder to store all medical documents in one place. Use dividers or tabs to separate sections such as medical history, test results, medication lists, appointment notes, and insurance documents. This can also be done electronically, although keeping paper copies helps—you will be surprised at how antiquated some systems can be. Within this storage, create a list that includes the names, contact information, and specialties of all the healthcare providers involved in your loved one's care. Include primary care physicians, specialists, therapists, and any other relevant professionals. It may be helpful to also keep a log to document any changes in symptoms or observations about your loved one's health. Note dates, descriptions of symptoms, severity, and any factors that may have influenced the symptoms. This information can help healthcare providers understand patterns and make more informed decisions.

Medication Management. Medication plays a crucial role in managing many chronic, degenerative diseases, including Alzheimer's disease, Parkinson's disease, and ALS. Although there are no medications that can stop neurocognitive conditions, there are medications that can slow disease progression. Medication can first and foremost help manage disease symptoms. Specific meds are geared toward treating certain symptoms. For a neurodegenerative disease, for instance, you would want a medication that improves memory. Oftentimes, a combination of medicines is prescribed. Medication is typically seen as complementary to other types of therapies or as part of a broader treatment plan.

Medication can also help with behavioral and psychological symptoms. Many loved ones who are suffering from an incurable disease experience symptoms like depression, anxiety, agitation, aggression, and hallucinations. These mood-related disorders are sometimes caused by the disease itself or are a secondary effect of coping with the knowledge of losing control over life. Medications such as antidepressants, antipsychotics, and anti-anxiety drugs can help manage these symptoms and help to improve the quality of life and the caregiving process.

Medications can also help patients maintain their independence and for a longer period, which may sustain their ability to perform daily activities more effectively, such as dressing, bathing, and engaging in social interactions for a longer period. They might, but medications are not a magic bullet. Be prepared to help your loved one sleep. This can include melatonin or other sleep aids to promote better sleep patterns. Lack of sleep is a common symptom that often predates and then exacerbates a decline.

It is almost certain that sometimes your loved one is going to be on a lot of medication. Pharmaceuticals are not magic bullets, but they can be incredible tools to help individuals coping with decline. The meds mentioned here are often in addition to whatever medications your loved one may be taking to support their heart, lungs, cholesterol, diabetes, etc.

Finding the right balance of medication was a huge challenge for our family. Dad was on medications for a heart condition before he was ever diagnosed with Alzheimer's. Eventually, he was on up to fifteen pills a day to manage his condition as it progressed. I couldn't tell you what each medication did. It actually became a huge source of confusion and a big undertaking to make sure the right pills were taken at the right time. In the doctor's first efforts to manage his symptoms, Dad got very sick from one combination of medication the doctor gave him to slow the disease. He was still cognitively sharp enough that he (with our support) decided the quality of his life was more important and he stopped that course of treatment. This kind of balance is important to find and an example of the tough decisions that need to be made.

Our family would be the first to notice when something wasn't working with Dad. In the last year of his life, we'd observe something off on a monthly basis, if not more frequently. Sometimes we would wonder if the medicines were doing anything at all—he seemed out of it and low. How could it be worse without meds? We had to clarify the purpose of each drug and try to understand if it was serving its purpose.

We not only had to know what medication he was on, but when to administer it. Always clarify with your provider what happens if a medication is missed, so you know what to do in the event that happens. It probably will. My mom had the foresight to work with our local pharmacy to make "pill packs" for him so he could pop one open for a given time of day and take those pills at once. This worked for a few months until the packs became too challenging to open. She then had to administer each pill to him. She also had to make sure he was able to sip water and swallow each pill. On occasion, we would find wet pills on the floor. Other times he would forget a pill was in his mouth and start going about his business, leaving it to get stuck or contra-indicate with another substance. Taking meds turned into a thirty-minute ordeal, three times a day.

Emergencies. When caregiving, always expect the unexpected. The unpredictability of a decline can mean more visits to the emergency room than you would expect. When supporting a loved one who is losing their faculties, it can be hard to know from their communication what constitutes an emergency and what does not. My friend Kate watched her mom indicate she was having trouble breathing, pointing to her chest, taking shallow breaths, and turning red in the face. She called an ambulance. The paramedics came, gave her oxygen immediately, and transported Kate and her mom to the hospital, where it appeared to have been a false alarm. Kate's mom was having an anxiety attack. There was no way for Kate to interpret these symptoms, so she did the only thing she could to get an answer.

The disease your loved one is dealing with can also demand emergency visits. My friend Jake supported his father, John, who had Parkinson's, and his mom, Kathy, the primary caretaker as his dad's condition deteriorated. Late one evening, John, who was in his early sixties, began experiencing severe chest pain and shortness of breath. Kathy helped him into their car and drove as quickly and safely as she could to the nearest hospital, where Jake met them. Upon arriving at the emergency room, Kathy rushed inside, explaining to the receptionist that her husband was experiencing severe chest pain and that he had Parkinson's. They were quickly triaged due to the severity of John's symptoms. The nurse took his vitals and asked about his medical history, paying close attention to the medications he was taking. John's tremors and stiffness made it difficult for him to speak clearly, but Mary was there to provide the necessary information. The emergency room doctor then tried to determine if John was having a heart attack. They moved him to a treatment room, where he was hooked up to a heart monitor. John's Parkinson's symptoms, such as his tremors and difficulty moving, made it harder for the staff to perform some of the tests. After what felt like an eternity, the doctor returned with the test results. John had experienced severe angina, but, thankfully, not a heart attack. They explained that his Parkinson's medication might have contributed to the chest pain and that they would need to adjust his treatment plan. The next day, a neurologist consulted with them to review the Parkinson's medications and ensure that any adjustments would not exacerbate John's symptoms.

While the outcome was a relief in the sense that John had not had a heart attack, it raised an important consideration. Now that it was clear from his experience that his medications were having negative effects, it was up to Mary and Jake to ensure John's care team knew of his reactions to his meds. That information was not necessarily going to be shared if they did not follow up.

Sometimes emergencies really are emergencies. Our dad had been experiencing flu-like symptoms and disorientation for a few days. One night, his vomiting was so severe that my sister and Mom drove him to the hospital. When he arrived, his speech was slurred, and he was still sick to his stomach. When they got him into a triage room, the nurses and physicians quickly realized he was having a neurologic issue. A scan found significant fluid around his brain. He was suffering from a subdural hematoma. Within six hours, he was going in for emergency brain surgery. This event happened before dad was diagnosed with Alzheimer's, but it shaped how our family responded to Dad's symptoms during his decline.

Trust in the Medical System. Being a caregiver means being asked to put a lot of trust in the medical system. This can be scary and, at times, infuriating. The reality is that there will be countless doctors, medications, appointments, and procedures, and sometimes the purpose of those visits will seem unclear. It will be draining to make the time for all these people and places, and it will be hard to not get the answers you seek from providers. Many degenerative illnesses come with so many unknowns that medical professionals can only do their best with the information they have.

There are plenty of reasons why it can be hard to trust our medical system. It is complicated and confusing, and not user friendly. Trying to understand health insurance, and which doctors to see, and what treatments you need, can feel overwhelming when you're primarily concerned for someone who is ailing. There are unexpected medical bills and high costs, even with insurance. These add to the frustration, make people question the value of care, and lead to a lot of stress and mistrust.

Past negative experiences can play a role in trust. If you or your loved one has been misdiagnosed, had a medical error, or felt rushed by a doctor who didn't take the time to listen (which happens all the time), it is hard to forget those experiences. Poor communication, where doctors use complicated medical terms or give conflicting opinions, can add to the burden.

Another pain point is that the medical system is not equal for all people. Language barriers, financial barriers, and discrimination plague medical care. There are issues with access and fairness. Many people face long waits for appointments, or they might not have access to good healthcare because of where they live, their income, or their background.

Systemic problems, such as bureaucracy and frequent changes in healthcare policies or providers, can disrupt continuity of care and create a sense of instability. Negative media coverage of medical scandals and the spread of misinformation also contribute to public distrust.

My own trust in the medical system was shaken during one of Dad's trips to the emergency room. He had been living in an Alzheimer's focused long-term care facility for about a month when his behavior became a cause for concern. He told one of the nurses there that he no longer wanted to live. He struck another patient. He was deemed a potential danger to himself and others and was sent to a hospital emergency room, where it was determined he required a geriatric psychiatric evaluation at a third facility (that had a geriatric psych ward) before he could return to his long-term care home. But the hospital did not believe that he qualified for a geriatric psych evaluation—he was not over sixty-five—and would not transfer him to the third facility. He was taken off the waiting list for transfer, without our family being informed, and kept in a general inpatient area where he shared a room with another patient for two weeks. The general hospital wanted to discharge him because he seemed calm and affable, but the long-term care facility would not take him back without the psych evaluation. While his visit started out as a few days' stay, it turned into a few weeks. He was in limbo at what was supposed to be one of the top medical facilities in the United States.

After about three weeks, Dad had an episode. He tried to leave the hospital and was physical with the nurses who tried to stop him. He lashed out with his arms to stop the nurses from touching him. He was put in full-body restraints and tied to his bed like a criminal. The restraints stayed on while he slept, which is a legal violation of patient's rights. Finally, the hospital understood it had done him an immense disservice by not getting him the psych evaluation, but seeing him in that bed, first in restraints and then in what appeared to be an adult crib, was heartbreaking and left me with disdain for that hospital. It is important to always remember that, in general, medical professionals and caregivers are both well-intentioned and doing the best they can at their jobs, but there are bound to be bumps on every medical journey.

Care Planning. We first talked about planning in Chapter 3. Here we'll add some details around healthcare planning, which is done in conjunction with a patient and a care team, or a patient navigator. It allows your loved one's providers to understand your family's priorities in their care. Sometimes providers take matters into their own hands, but it is critical that you write down what *you* and your loved one want. Do they have end-of-life care plans? Do they have a DNR order ("do not resuscitate" in the event of cardiac arrest)? Care planning aims to ensure that all aspects of an individual's physical, mental, and social well-being are addressed. Here are the key components and steps involved in the care planning process:

- Assessment. The first step is to conduct a thorough assessment of the individual's current health status, medical history, functional abilities, and psychosocial needs. This assessment may involve input from healthcare professionals, family members, and the individual themselves. The process is often led by a care navigator.

- Goal Setting. These are established based on your priorities, but typically they should be measurable, realistic, and aligned with your loved one's preferences and values. Examples of goals may include managing pain, improving mobility, extending quality of life, enjoying sugar, or enhancing time with friends. The goals are often not just a specific medical goal but ways to support daily life.

- Care Plan Development: This is actually like a living document. It outlines the strategies, interventions, and services that care providers and your family will employ to support your goals. It includes details such as medication management, supportive therapies, dietary considerations, social activities, and any necessary equipment or assistive devices that the family needs. The care is regularly reviewed and updated as needed by changes to your loved one.

- Care Coordination. All healthcare providers, therapists, pharmacists, and family members involved in your loved one's care should be aware of and aligned with the care plan. It involves clear communication, sharing of information, and collaboration among the various members of the care team.

- Review and Modify: Care plans are constantly changing and need to be updated to reflect changes in your loved one's condition, preferences, or goals. Ongoing communication and feedback from the individual, caregivers, and healthcare providers help inform these modifications. There may come a point when your loved one's opinions keep changing, and you will have to use your best judgment and rely on their written wishes.

A whole book could be written about navigating the healthcare system. The TL;DR is that there will be key areas of healthcare that may surprise you, confuse you, and disappoint you. Care planning will help you deal with the challenges of meeting the needs of your loved one. Healthcare in the traditional sense—doctors, nurses, hospitals—is a critical resource and a time-consuming part of caregiving, but it will probably not give you the answers you need as a caregiver. Each patient is incredibly distinct. Use these care providers and medical visits as a resource, always keeping your loved one's quality of life in mind.

CHAPTER 7

Digital Tools

DIGITAL LIFE WAS A PAIN POINT FOR OUR FAMILY when my dad got sick. When he could no longer leave the house independently, we lived in fear of what he might accidentally post on Facebook as he mindlessly (literally) scrolled his phone. Those fears were realized one day in 2022 when I logged on to Facebook to see that he had posted a selfie of his nose and asked his followers for help in deciding when to run for president. We think he was referring to a local board of electors race, but the world will never know.

After that incident, we subtlety tried to delete his Facebook, but somehow the app would find a way back on to his phone. Dad clung to his computer and his phone for a long time. We eventually got him an Alzheimer's-friendly mobile, which meant he could click on our pictures and it would call us. This phone took the apps out of his hands while alleviating his stress from dealing with numeracy and small touch-screen buttons. He kept his de-activated iPhone so he could scroll through pictures of his family and remember happier times. In moments when he would space out or get lost in frustration, photos of family and his dog would inevitably bring him back.

He would laugh his full belly laugh when we showed him a photo of his grandson making a goofy face.

There were also a lot of painful calls and three-minute voicemails in which the only audible words were "help me, I'm stuck." We think he meant he was stuck in his own mind, but we really couldn't tell. Those messages remain on my voicemail log. Now that he's gone, I can't bring myself to delete them, despite how painful some are—reminders of the pain he was in and how he was no longer himself. But they let me hear his voice, however strained it had become. And I still have the voicemail he left to wish me a happy birthday the year before he died. That is one I will cherish.

Digital tools can be the devil and also your friend. They can help organize care coordination, support you, support your loved one, and sustain your memories.

If you're a millennial, chances are that technology is an integral part of your daily routine, shaping how you communicate, work, entertain yourself, and manage various aspects of your life. Your smartphone is probably the most essential tool you own. It's your connection to social media, where platforms like Facebook, Instagram, and TikTok allow you to share your life, stay updated with friends, and engage with a constant stream of content. You scroll through your feeds, liking, commenting, and sharing posts that resonate with you, making social media a central hub for your interactions. It's your gateway to the world.

In most professional lives, technology is also indispensable. Whether you're working remotely or in an office, tools like Slack, Zoom, and Google Workspace keep colleagues connected and projects on track. The rise of the gig economy has given you the flexibility to take on freelance work through platforms like Upwork and Fiverr, or driving for Uber and Lyft when you need extra income.

Streaming services have become the primary source of entertainment for many. Millions of people have "cut the cord" and swapped traditional TV and radio for the flexibility of Netflix, Hulu, and Spotify. These platforms let anyone watch their favorite shows or movies, and listen to music at their convenience on any device. The ability to binge-watch a series or create personalized playlists means entertainment is always tailored to your preferences and schedule.

Shopping is also digital. Online platforms like Amazon have become the first option for many who are purchasing. The convenience of browsing, comparing prices, reading reviews, and having items delivered to your door is unmatched. This digital shopping experience saves time and often money, making it a preferred choice over physical stores.

Even financial management is now digital. Checkbook ledgers seem to have become a thing of the past, thanks to mobile banking apps letting you check your balance, transfer money, and pay bills with a few taps. Investment apps like Robinhood and Acorns make investing accessible, even if you're a novice.

Technology plays a supportive role in your health and fitness. Wearable devices such as Fitbits or Apple Watches track your physical activity, sleep patterns, and your heart rate. Fitness apps guide people through workouts and track progress, while meditation apps like Headspace help you manage stress and maintain mental wellbeing. Telehealth services have also made it easier to consult with healthcare professionals without leaving your home.

When it comes to travel, technology simplifies everything. Booking flights and accommodations through apps like Expedia and Airbnb is quick and easy, often offering better deals than traditional travel agencies. Navigation apps like Google Maps ensure people never get lost, providing real-time traffic updates and route suggestions.

Lifelong learning is another area where you leverage technology. Online platforms like Coursera, Udemy, and Khan Academy offer courses on virtually any topic, allowing you to expand your knowledge and skills at your own pace. You might also listen to podcasts and attend webinars to stay informed and inspired.

Why this long list of the uses of technology? The reality is that technology can play a huge role in caregiving across these dimensions. Researchers have found that the millennials generation's use of technology is integral to its experience of caregiving. And millennials use technology differently than earlier generations: they prefer texts for private communications and alter their social media use once becoming caregivers due to feelings of envy over others' enjoyment. Baby Boomers feel more connected through Zoom.[10]

How Can Digital Tools Help?

Digital tools can play a significant role in streamlining caregiver tasks and making caregiving more efficient and organized. These tools are generally accessible, cost-effective, and time-efficient, making them suitable for a caregivers' busy lifestyle.

Digital tools can help out in the following ways:

- Care Coordination and Communication. Digital tools can keep you in touch with family members, healthcare professionals, and other caregivers involved in the care of an individual. Online calendars, messaging apps, and care management platforms allow caregivers to share information, coordinate schedules, and communicate updates easily. These are probably pretty familiar to many folks who are already guided by Google Calendar or Outlook and the other daily trackers that keep us moving from place to place.

- Medication Management. There are various medication reminder apps and pill organizer apps available that send reminders for medication doses, provide information about medications, and allow caregivers to record medication adherence. Subscription services can also make sure medications are delivered right to your home so that you don't have to go to the pharmacy every month. Dad took about fifteen pills a day, at three different times, and not always the same dose every day. For our family, subscribing to a medication delivery service was essential.

- Health Monitoring. Devices such as blood pressure monitors, glucose meters, or wearable fitness trackers provide real-time health data that can be tracked and shared with healthcare professionals, helping to identify any potential issues or trends. Millions of people are already hooked up to Fitbits, Apple watches, and similar fitness-tracking devices. It can be beneficial to use these apps and create an account on your phone to view your loved ones' vitals on a regular basis. Some doctors will ask for regular check-ins and these tools can make it easy.

- Digital Documentation and Information Storage. Using cloud-based storage or digital document management systems, caregivers can securely store and access important documents, medical records, insurance information, and legal documents related to caregiving. This streamlines information retrieval and reduces the risk of physical document loss. Digital tools allow caregivers to maintain and access electronic health records, and to store important medical information, test results, and treatment plans, making them easier to access and share when necessary. Downloading an app on your phone that can scan documents directly to password-protected cloud storage can be a big help.

- Caregiver Support and Education. Online resources, support groups, and educational materials are readily available through websites and mobile apps. These platforms offer valuable information, tips, and guidance on various caregiving topics, helping caregivers navigate their roles more effectively. There are many free resources online that can support the mental health of caregivers. There are also numerous free courses on how to become a caregiver. All of the support groups our family participated in were online. Same for almost everyone I have talked to in the past few years. Naturally, it makes getting support easier. You just have to set aside an hour and a half for the group, without additional commuting time each way.

- Remote Monitoring and Telehealth. Telehealth platforms enable remote consultations with healthcare professionals, reducing the need for in-person visits. This can be particularly beneficial for caregivers who face challenges with transportation or have difficulty bringing the care recipient to healthcare appointments. We would not have been able to care for Dad as effectively had we not used Telehealth. It allowed him to go "alone" to appointments. Online therapy allowed us to take care of ourselves without worrying about leaving him alone all day.

- Emergency Response Systems. Digital tools such as personal emergency response systems (PERS) or mobile apps can provide immediate assistance in case of emergencies. These tools allow caregivers to quickly alert emergency services or designated contacts in the event of a medical crisis or safety concern.

Digital Resources for Caregivers

There are several online resources available to support caregivers. These can provide caregivers with information, support, and connections to other caregivers facing similar challenges. It's important to evaluate the credibility and relevance of the information provided from these sources, and you'll still want to consult with healthcare professionals for personalized advice and guidance. As you will see, none of these resources are catered toward young, millennial caregivers. However, they still have helpful information.

Here are some reputable websites and platforms that provide valuable information, tools, and support for caregivers:

- Caregiver Action Network (CAN). Offers a wide range of resources, including educational materials, online support groups, and a caregiver toolbox with practical tips and resources. Their website provides information on various caregiving topics and hosts webinars and educational events. https://www.caregiveraction.org/
- Family Caregiver Alliance (FCA). Offers a wealth of resources for caregivers, including fact sheets, online support groups, and educational materials. Their website provides information on different health conditions, caregiver rights, and practical advice for managing caregiving responsibilities. https://www.caregiver.org/
- AARP Caregiving Resource Center. AARP provides a comprehensive caregiving resource center with articles, tips, and tools to support caregivers. Their website offers information on topics such as legal and financial planning, caregiver stress, and navigating the healthcare system. https://www.aarp.org/caregiving/
- National Alliance for Caregiving. A non-profit organization dedicated to supporting family caregivers. Their website provides resources, research findings, and information on caregiving policy issues. They also offer a Caregiver Resource Directory to help caregivers locate local support services. https://www.caregiving.org/
- Well Spouse Association. Provides support for spousal caregivers. Their website offers online support groups, resource articles, and information on respite programs for spousal caregivers. https://wellspouse.org/
- Lotsa Helping Hands: An online caregiving coordination platform that helps caregivers organize support, communicate with

family and friends, and coordinate tasks. The platform allows caregivers to create a caregiving community and streamline caregiving responsibilities. https://lotsahelpinghands.com/

These mobile apps may be of help:

- CareZone. A comprehensive app designed for caregivers to organize and manage various aspects of caregiving. It allows you to create and share a care calendar, track medications, store medical records, take notes, and set reminders for appointments and tasks. The app also offers a journal feature for recording observations and a secure messaging function for communication with the care team.

- CaringBridge. A platform that allows caregivers to create a private website or journal to provide updates on their loved one's health. It enables family and friends to stay informed, leave supportive messages, and coordinate support. The app includes a planner feature for organizing tasks, a journal for recording updates, and a messaging function.

- MyDirectives. An app that helps caregivers and individuals create and store advance care directives and medical preferences. It allows users to document their healthcare wishes, including end-of-life decisions, and securely share these directives with healthcare providers, family members, and caregivers. The app also includes emergency contact information and a feature for organizing important documents.

- Caregiver: Developed by Care.com, this app helps families and caregivers manage care for loved ones. It includes features such as a shared calendar, task list, messaging, and photo sharing. The app allows for easy coordination and communication among family members and caregivers involved in the care of a loved one.

There are also many disease-specific organizations that can provide resources tailored to the ailment of your loved one. These might be the Alzheimer's Association, the Parkinson's Foundation, the Susan G. Komen Breast Cancer Foundation, the American Cancer Society, the American Heart Association, and the list goes on.

The Good and the Bad of Online Tools

Online resources offer significant advantages, starting with accessibility and convenience. It allows unprecedented access to a vast range of health information from anywhere at any time, which is especially beneficial for those in remote or underserved areas. Access to online content saves time and eliminates the need for physical visits to libraries or healthcare providers. Medical journals and health organizations, patient forums, and news articles can all be accessed via the internet, providing a comprehensive view of health topics and the latest updates on advancements and research findings. This can be incredibly empowering to caregivers, allowing them to learn about their loved one's conditions, treatments, and preventative measures. It leads to more informed decisions and enables them to advocate during medical appointments. Online communities offer support networks where individuals can share experiences, seek advice, and find emotional support from others with similar experiences.

The internet is also a rabbit hole. The quality and reliability of information can be questionable, if not rife with inaccurate or misleading health information and non-expert opinions. It can be challenging to distinguish credible sources from unreliable ones. With the growth of artificial intelligence, this will probably increase. The overwhelming volume of information can also make it difficult to find relevant and accurate data, and conflicting information from different sources can cause confusion and uncertainty.

Searches on the internet often lead to confirmation bias, which means people are more likely to only read articles that reinforce what they are already looking for. This wasn't the case with our family. We knew that there was only one eventual outcome, so we weren't "looking for a fix." If you are clinging to hopes of a miraculous cure, you should approach the internet

Online health research often provides general information. It may or may not apply to the individual circumstances of your loved one. Making your own diagnosis and treatment plan can lead to incorrect or delayed medical care.

Researching health information online can also expose you to privacy risks. Websites sometimes track search activities and collect personal information without consent. Participating in online forums or support groups might inadvertently reveal personal health information if proper privacy measures are not in place.

To maximize the benefits and minimize the risks of online health research, it is crucial to use reputable sources, verify information with healthcare professionals, and be mindful of privacy practices while researching health topics online.

Here are some steps to effectively conduct research online:

• Identify Reliable Sources. When you go to the internet to explore your loved one's condition, start with reputable sources, especially those affiliated with national governments or research institutes. Other trusted sources include government health agencies (Centers for Disease Control and Prevention, National Institutes of Health, and the UK's National Health Service), reputable medical organizations (Mayo Clinic, WebMD), and academic institutions. These websites often offer detailed articles, fact sheets, symptom checkers, treatment options, and other relevant resources. If you want to delve deeper into the scientific literature, you can search online databases such as PubMed,

Google Scholar, or the Cochrane Library. These platforms provide access to a wide range of scholarly articles, research papers, and clinical studies related to health conditions.

• Evaluate the Credibility of Information. When you encounter new health information, try to assess the credibility and accuracy of the source. You can look for particular clues. For example, look for references to scientific studies, medical experts, and peer-reviewed publications. Be particularly cautious of websites that lack references to scientific studies or only identify alternative treatments. Many treatments that are recommended by conventional medicine have been through decades or at least years of scientific study. Most alternative treatments have not gone through the same process and will not have the same level of details to back up their claims.

• Check Out Patient Forums. Online patient forums and support groups can offer valuable information and personal experiences related to specific health conditions. This can provide insight into what the experience may be like if your family pursues a particular course of action. You may learn novel things about medication or a course of action being recommended to you. However, read these forums with a grain of salt. People on these platforms are sharing experiences from their individual perspectives. They are not trained medical professionals, and they have their biases or rationale for health decisions. The best option would be to use these sources as a supplementary resource rather than a definitive source.

• Stay Updated with Current Research. For many medical conditions, scientific developments are constantly unfolding. In 2024, the United States Food and Drug Administration approved new treatment options for ALS and Alzheimer's. Stay informed by following reputable medical journals, news outlets, or academic institutions. These groups often publish articles or press releases summarizing new findings and developments. However, do not hold out unrealistic hope that a new research study will be available in time to help your loved one. The turnaround time for a new trial to market can be extremely long. There are very specific parameters for eligibility in trials.

• Talk to Healthcare Professionals. While online research can provide valuable information, it's important to remember that healthcare professionals are the most reliable sources of personalized advice. Discuss your findings with healthcare providers to obtain professional guidance and ensure the information aligns with your specific situation. Online research should supplement, and not replace, the professional advice your family is getting. We followed the advice of our Dad's clinicians rather than what internet naturalists said in terms of how to approach nutritional needs. That being said, we are all constantly online, and it is natural to use the vast resources we have at our fingertips.

How to Identify Misinformation

Misinformation refers to information that is either intentionally false or untrue when taken out of context. Identifying misinformation online is crucial for making informed decisions about your loved one's care and to your own mental health and well-being. To start, always check the source of the information. Trustworthy sources include government websites, reputable news organizations, and accredited educational institutions. Look into the author's credentials to ensure they are experts in the field. Cross-referencing information with multiple reliable sources and using fact-checking websites like Snopes or FactCheck.org can also help verify accuracy. These resources are particularly helpful for general information but may not be helpful for your caregiving experience.

Pay attention to the language used. Reliable content is usually presented in a neutral, unbiased manner and cites credible sources. Because misinformation may just be outdated information, make sure the information is current by checking the publication date, as outdated data can be misleading. Be skeptical of simplistic solutions to complex issues, and seek out content that offers a balanced, nuanced perspective. Trustworthy sources often include disclaimers and transparent editorial standards, so look for these indicators. It's also important to recognize your own biases and avoid only seeking information that confirms your pre-existing beliefs. Analyze the website's design and domain—professional, well-maintained sites with secure HTTPS connections are generally more reliable. Consider the intent behind the content. If it seems to be pushing an agenda or trying to sell something, be cautious. Obviously, a website selling bananas is going to tell you bananas are good for you. Less obviously, a website that advertises itself as a clinician's guide to brain health may tell you bananas are good for you and not mention that it takes money from banana producers. Both should be met with healthy skepticism.

Social Media Dos and Don'ts

Social media can be an amazing way to stay connected with family, friends, and your broader network on your caregiving journey. It offers a valuable platform for connecting with other caregivers. Through groups and forums, you can share experiences, seek advice, and find comfort in knowing you're not alone. There are hundreds of support groups on Facebook and websites like AgingCare.com that are specifically designed for people who are caregiving for someone with a particular type of ailment. Many of these support groups are full of individuals who are likely in the Boomer generation (or older). Boomers tend to be more active on Facebook and online forums, so it may not feel like you are surrounded by peers, but there can still be comradery in shared experience.

Millennials tend to be more active on social media platforms other than Facebook.[11] If you are an active user of Instagram, X, or LinkedIn, you follow relevant organizations, healthcare providers, advocacy groups, or researchers on those platforms. These connections are likely to share valuable information, educational resources, and updates related to caregiving and specific health conditions you are interested in. These organizations tend to be active on social media and will reply to comments on their posts. Similarly, you might find micro-influencers who have caregiving recommendations for anything from nurses to child psychologists to relevant nonprofits.

On the downside, social media can sometimes lead to information overload, with conflicting advice and unreliable sources that can cause confusion and stress. Similar to what we noted about verifying your sources, take what you see on social media from individuals who are not affiliated with a reputable institution with caution. These are opinions, not facts. Oftentimes, individuals on social media are paid to focus on particular resources or courses of treatment.

Social media can also be challenging for caregivers who are constantly exposed to the seemingly perfect lives of peers who are not caregiving. I know three caregivers who deleted their Instagrams and Facebook pages because viewing other happy family lives was just too much to process during caregiving. Only you know the right balance of using social media for your personal enjoyment and caregiving journey, but balancing these pros and cons is essential to make the most of social media as a caregiver.

Summing It Up

Digital tools are ubiquitous in our way of life. The TL;DR is that caregivers can rely on digital tools to support their caregiving journey. It makes sense to rely on tools you are already comfortable with and identify apps that feel user-friendly based on your own experience of digital space. Think of digital tools as resources that can make your life easier, facilitate research, and help you connect with others. Many of the special people I have met through the caregiving community operate their own social media spaces. These can be very helpful to caregivers. My family also connected with individuals through online forums who offered their stories to us as caregivers and later agreed for them to be shared in this book.

CHAPTER 8

Financial Realities

M Y DAD ALWAYS PAID HIS BILLS ON TIME. HE HAD one credit card that he paid off each month, and often when we ate out, he preferred to pay cash. About a year before he was diagnosed with Alzheimer's, my sister noticed Visa sending him a lot more mail. He didn't have a Visa, as far as we knew. The mail from Visa went into the trash. She thought it was junk.

A few months went by, and Dad became increasingly absent minded with his phone. My sister was holding it one day when we were out and saw an automated message pop up: "Your payment of $3,346.87 for account ending in XX91 is due on 3/7/21."

Dad had a four-figure balance on a credit-card account we had never seen before. As it turned out, he was long overdue. My sister's eyes bulged out when she saw by how much.

This started our family's investigation into Dad's finances. He not only had opened up a new credit card, but he had auto-subscribed to multiple media outlets and subscription services with that new credit card, leading to hundreds of charges a month. In total, Dad had debts of $14,000 across multiple accounts. His retirement savings had been accessed and were nearly depleted. Automatic payments became his enemy.

It took months to figure out what all the charges were and pay off his credit card. It took months more to close the card. It's very difficult to actually convince a financial services company that an adult who is not institutionalized wants to close a credit card. Our economy thrives on credit and debt, and creditors live for people like my dad who forget to pay their bills (or can't) and rack up thousands of dollars in interest.

Despite having no sense of money, time, or autonomy, Dad was tanking his perfect credit score, too. The icing on the cake was when financial representatives would ask to talk to him before he could close his account. Their policies and procedures precluded them from taking my word or my sister's word that Dad was incapable of making financial decisions and we were acting as his representative. Eventually, we put him on the phone. He would say hello and then unceremoniously end the conversation by putting the phone down on the counter without hanging up, likely because he forgot he was on the phone in the first place. When my sister or I would resume the conversation with the financial representative, it took willpower to not say "I told ya so."

The credit card was the tip of the iceberg. We knew we needed to shut down Dad's accounts because he could no longer manage his finances. Because it's the 2020s, many of our family's bills were automated: phone, cable, internet, electric. Many of those automatic payments required password logins to change or reset. In order to change a password, you need to answer security questions about the account holder. When the account holder has no recollection of the account, you are up a creek. My sister, brother, and I did our best. It took nearly a full year to cancel or change accounts. Some providers refused to make changes without an affidavit from a health-care provider, a death notice (which we obviously did not have), a notarized letter, or a blood sample—kidding about the last one, but it felt that way. The time we spent on this was astounding. Financial swings are a brutal reality of caring for an ailing loved one. In an ideal world, the person you are caring for has the financial means to contribute to their care and adapt to lifestyle changes. In other instances, their resources will be limited, and you'll have to evaluate your own financial reality and how much you can contribute.

Losses can come in different ways. If the person you are caring for worked before their illness, there will probably be a loss of income. If you're now a caregiver and can no longer work outside the home, there may be a reduction in how much you can contribute. There are also new expenses: out-of-pocket medical costs, supplemental therapies, additional transportation, new clothes if their condition is impacting their size—it all adds up.

There may be additional expenses your loved one has incurred without your knowledge, as was the case with my dad. One Monday in March, seventy-two bagels showed up at my parent's house. That's over $100 worth of bagels. We had no idea how they got there. After a couple of hours of investigation, we realized Dad had signed up through Facebook for a monthly bagel subscription. Six dozen bagels the first Monday of the month. The subscription was canceled. We had frozen bagels for weeks.

Caregiving is expensive. There is frankly no financially neutral way to support a loved one. Some of the more common caregiving costs include:

- Medical Expenses. Caregivers are often fronting the money for medical expenses, including doctor visits, medications, medical equipment, and specialized treatments. These costs can add up significantly, especially if the care recipient has a chronic or complex medical condition.

- Personal Care Expenses. This includes the costs of daily needs such as food, clothing, personal hygiene products, and household supplies for the care recipient. Caregivers may need to purchase these items on behalf of the person they are caring for. It sounds silly, but there may also be times during the caregiving journey when you decide to spend more to protect your mental health, or the well-being of your loved one. Going to the grocery store became excruciatingly painful for me and my dad. We would arrive as usual, and he would become fixated on finding a particular item, like Cap'n Crunch All Red Berries. When he inevitably could not find this cereal, he would pace the cereal aisle in agitation. Once he actually sat on the floor of the grocery store. We laugh-cried. It was terrible. Another time, he became so frustrated with a slow cashier that he attempted to leave without paying for the three bags of candy in his hand. I decided to start ordering groceries to be delivered to his home. This increased our grocery bill by about 10 percent a week.

- Home Health or Facility Costs. In some instances, caregivers may need to hire professional caregivers to assist with their loved ones. These services can be expensive and may include hourly rates, overnight care, or live-in arrangements. At some point, it may be necessary to move your loved one to a residential facility like a nursing home, acute care, or memory care facility. The Genworth 2020 Cost of Care Survey reports that the national median cost for in-home care services is around $4,300 per month for homemaker services and $4,400 for home health aide services. Assisted living facilities have a median cost of about $4,300 per month, while a semi-private room in a nursing home can cost a median of $7,756 per month. Given inflation and the rising cost of healthcare, these costs are likely to increase.

- Transportation Costs. Caregivers often need to get the care recipient to medical appointments, therapy sessions, or social activities. Expenses may include fuel costs, parking fees, or public transportation fares. In instances where the loved one must go to an adult day care or attend appointments that you cannot take them to, there are transportation services available through senior-services organizations, which may help to offset these costs. Transportation was a huge trigger point for our family. Dad was incredibly aggressive in the car. He had always been the driver of the family and would still try to get in the driver's seat. If we got him to the passenger's seat without a fuss, he would often try to grab the steering wheel or change gears if he got frustrated with the route or traffic. It was dangerous to drive with him. We started using a service to take him places whenever possible.

- Lost Wages and Reduced Work Hours. Many caregivers need to reduce their work hours or leave their jobs altogether to provide care, resulting in a loss of income and potential career opportunities. This can have long-term financial implications. Unpaid caregiving responsibilities often impact a caregiver's employment. About seven in ten caregivers report making work-related adjustments due to their caregiving responsibilities, such as reducing work hours, taking a leave of absence, or quitting their job altogether.

- Home Modifications. In some cases, caregivers decide to make modifications to their loved one's home to accommodate the needs of the care recipient. This can include installing ramps, grab bars, or making other accessibility modifications. It can be costly. We got automatic sinks installed, which meant the water bill could go up on a monthly basis, but we were more likely to avoid a flood if the top was left open for an indeterminate amount of time.

- Legal and Financial Assistance. Caregivers may need advice to manage their loved one's affairs. This can involve attorney fees, accountant fees, or expenses related to establishing power of attorney or guardianship.

- Emotional and Physical Health Expenses. Caregiving can take a toll on the caregiver's emotional and physical well-being. Costs related to stress management, therapy, or medical care for the caregiver themselves may be incurred. Many organizations provide free support. Your loved one's clinical team can help point you in the right direction, as can the local bureau on aging, or the nonprofit associated with your loved one's disease.

If you weren't overwhelmed before, the financial realities of the caregiver role make even the savviest person squirm. If I'm being super honest, the thought of budgeting has made my head spin from the time I was sixteen and spent every babysitting paycheck at TJ Maxx.

I wish someone had really hammered home to my family the financial realities of a long-term degenerative illness. The burden to people and society of caregiving is vast and growing. According to the National Alliance for Caregiving and AARP, at any given time there are approximately fifty-three million unpaid caregivers in the United States responsible for adults or children with special needs. Unpaid caregivers are worth *a lot* in terms of their economic and social contributions. In 2020 alone, the collective value of all that unpaid caregiving amounted to a staggering $470 billion.

So, what can you do? Let's break it down step by step.

Step 1. Check your loved one's finances

Start by understanding where your loved one stands financially. Figure out what comes in on the plus side—income, savings, and investments—and also look into expenses such as debts, home loans,

outstanding credit card bills, and any other ongoing financial commitments. Cancel ongoing subscriptions to activities they can no
longer pursue, like club or gym memberships. The expenses may
change over time, but it's valuable to know your starting point. This
will help you see what resources are available and where there may
be gaps. It can also be helpful to make a list of any property, real
estate, or other assets that your loved one has because may need to
sell or rent to raise funds.

Review your loved one's health insurance, long-term care insurance, and any other policies that could help with costs. The US
health insurance system is about as complicated as things get, but
more recent healthcare laws have created requirements for transpar-
ency in coverage and for more disclosure by insurance companies.
Use this to your advantage. Call the health insurance company
and have it review the relevant policy. If your loved one does not
have private health insurance, and meets a particular age threshold (sixty-five), they are eligible for Medicare (federal insurance for
older adults). However, Medicare is only required to pay for hospital coverage (Medicare Part A) and other select services (Medicare
Part B) unless your loved one has chosen to pay for a supplemental
Medicare plan, known as Medicare Part C. Each state has information on its website and typically provides access to patient navigators
to help you select the best plan for you or your loved one. Use
these services to your advantage. If your loved one meets a disability
or income threshold, they are also eligible for the federal program
Medicaid, another source of insurance that varies by state. People
who are eligible for Medicare and Medicaid are known as dual eligible. Determining which program(s) your loved one can access can
be time-consuming up front, but enormously beneficial in terms of
cost. So take a close look at your parent's health insurance to see what
it covers and what it doesn't, and think about getting extra insurance
or a long-term care policy to help with specific needs or to give more

financial protection. Additional insurance programs such as long-term care coverage are something that your loved one may have a policy for.

Step 2. Find out what help is available

Look into options that may support you as a caregiver or your loved one as a patient. Particular programs to pay attention to fall into three buckets: employer benefits (if you are employed), insurance programs, and nonprofit options.

Bucket 1. Some employers offer benefits and support programs specifically designed to assist caregivers. These benefits are intended to help employees balance their work responsibilities with their caregiving responsibilities. Here are some common employer benefits for caregivers:

- Flexible Work Arrangements. Employers may offer flexible work options such as telecommuting, flexible hours, part-time schedules, or job sharing to accommodate the caregiving needs of their employees. This can help caregivers manage their caregiving responsibilities while still maintaining employment.
- Paid Time Off (PTO) and Family Leave. Some employers allow employees to take time away from work to care for a family member. This may include maternity or paternity leave, parental leave, or leave for caring for an ill family member.
- Employee Assistance Programs (EAP). EAPs are employer-sponsored programs that offer confidential counseling and support services to employees. These programs can provide resources and guidance on managing caregiving responsibilities and may offer referrals to community resources and support networks.

- Caregiver Support and Education. Employers may offer educational resources, workshops, or support groups specifically tailored to caregivers. These programs can provide information, training, and emotional support to help caregivers navigate their roles more effectively.
- Employee Wellness Programs. These may include resources and services that support caregivers' physical and mental health, such as stress management programs, counseling services, or wellness activities. These programs can help caregivers maintain their well-being while juggling their caregiving responsibilities.
- Employee Benefits. Some employers offer benefits packages that include insurance coverage for medical expenses, including those related to caregiving, such as dependent care coverage, long-term care insurance, or caregiver support services.

Bucket 2. Here are some common insurance benefits that may be available to caregivers. Also check out the government programs like Medicare, Medicaid, or benefits for veterans that can help pay for your parent's care.

- Health Insurance. Caregivers may be covered under their own health insurance plans, which can provide coverage for medical expenses related to their own health needs. It is important for caregivers to maintain their own health insurance coverage to address their personal healthcare needs.
- Dependent Coverage. Many health insurance plans provide coverage for dependents, including children or spouses. Depending on the policy, these plans may cover the medical expenses of the person receiving care, including doctor visits, hospital stays, medications, and treatments.
- Long-Term Care Insurance. Long-term care insurance is a specific type of insurance designed to cover the costs associated with

long-term care services, including home care, assisted living, and nursing home care. Some policies may also provide coverage for respite care, which allows caregivers to take a temporary break from their caregiving responsibilities.

- Disability Insurance. Disability insurance provides income replacement if the caregiver becomes unable to work due to a disability or injury. This can be helpful if the caregiver's ability to work and earn income is compromised due to caregiving responsibilities or other factors.
- Life Insurance. Life insurance policies provide financial protection to the beneficiaries in the event of the caregiver's death. The policy payout can be used to cover funeral expenses, outstanding debts, or provide financial support to the care recipient.

Bucket 3. There are several nonprofits and organizations that provide support and assistance to caregivers in managing their caregiving expenses. Here are a few examples:

- National Alliance for Caregiving (NAC). NAC is a nonprofit organization that offers resources, support, and advocacy for caregivers. It provides information on various caregiving topics and offer assistance in finding local resources, including financial assistance programs.
- Family Caregiver Alliance (FCA). FCA is a national nonprofit organization that provides support and resources to caregivers. It offers information on caregiving issues, online support groups, and a Family Care Navigator tool that helps locate local resources, including financial assistance programs.
- National Council on Aging (NCOA). NCOA is a nonprofit organization dedicated to improving the lives of older adults. It provides information and resources on caregiving, including financial assistance programs, benefits eligibility, and assistance with managing healthcare costs.

- Area Agencies on Aging (AAA). AAA is a network of organizations that provides services and support to older adults and caregivers at the local level. It can offer information on available resources, including financial assistance programs specific to the region or community.
- Local Nonprofit Organizations. Many communities have local nonprofits or community organizations that offer assistance and support to caregivers. These organizations may provide grants, respite care services, support groups, or other resources to help with caregiving expenses. Local senior centers or social service agencies can often provide information on these organizations.
- Disease-specific Organizations. Organizations like the Alzheimer's Association, American Cancer Society, or American Heart Association, along with their local chapters or affiliates, can provide assistance to caregivers.

The system of potential services is often unclear, and some may argue that it is deliberately vague so that people are less likely to utilize services available. You may spend extended periods of time trying to access programs you know that your loved one qualifies for. It's a good idea to talk to a financial planner or advisor who knows about taking care of older adults or planning for long-term care. They can help you figure out how your loved one's needs will affect your finances, look at your own financial situation, and come up with a plan that works for both of you. They can also help you with things like investing, planning for retirement, and dealing with taxes. A lawyer who knows elder law may also be helpful in figuring out what support is available and if your loved one qualifies. For some programs, a social worker or care advisor may be able to point you in the right direction and help you get the necessary paperwork to prove your eligibility.

Step 3. Make a budget

While you're planning for your loved one's care, make sure to think about your own finances, too. Consider how taking care of your loved one might affect your own money goals, plans for retirement, and career. It's important to find a balance between supporting your loved one and making sure you're financially secure. See Appendix for a helpful budgeting worksheet.

Medicare or Medicaid does not kick in until medical needs are severe. However, you may be able to get paid to be a caregiver for your loved one. Most states have a program that allows a family member to be a paid caregiver. The programs vary on a state-by-state basis. Check out your state's Medicaid website to understand the expectations (likely your loved one will need to be on Medicaid and already qualified for in-home healthcare).

Put together a detailed budget that covers all the costs of taking care of your loved one. This includes medical bills, prescriptions, changes to their home, help they might need at home, the cost of moving to assisted living or a nursing home, transportation, and anything else they need. Think about both short-term needs and what might come up down the road. In some ways, it's best to know up front both your family's priorities and what budget you are working with. For our family, it was critical that Dad stay living at home as long as possible, until he was literally a danger to himself or others. We made many physical adjustments to the house. Our family brought in therapists who could see him at home. These costs added up. Were they worth it at the time? Yes, every moment felt worth it, but in reality, we were often taking expensive steps that helped minimally. I am not discouraging you from using your resources, but it is important to have realistic expectations about how expensive supplemental support can be, and that there may be limited returns on that investment. When you are in the thick of caregiving, you will do pretty much anything within your power to support your loved one, but you will never know when taking an action how beneficial it may be and for how long it will work. Sometimes, when there is a financial cost, it's a challenge.

The other thing to keep in mind is the challenge of knowing how long to make your financial plan. You may be asking yourself, Am I budgeting for a year? Two years? Five? Ten? With degenerative conditions, it is very hard to know. Even some people who have planned extensively for retirement, worked their whole lives, and saved a lot of money spend all of their resources on care-related needs. It can be dangerous to assume that you are only planning for the short term in making decisions. Work with your healthcare team to get a sense of the potential horizon of your loved one's condition. Try to have a financial inflection point, some particular threshold—dollars in the bank, expenditures per month, or amount of debt—that will force a pivot in your care plan.

Step 4. Adapt the budget

A particularly brutal aspect of my family's situation was that some supplemental therapies were not covered by insurance. We would meet to weigh the pros and cons of something like occupational therapy to help dad's motor skills. We would agree to proceed in some instances, but within two months, notice there was no effect. Dad was coming home frustrated and depressed at his failure to grasp the therapy, and we were out of pocket a couple hundred dollars. On the flip side, Dad had always loved playing guitar. We hired a music therapist to come to the house and work with him. It was one of the things he most enjoyed each week. Even when he moved to a residential facility, he kept playing. We paid for that music therapist to visit him in his residential facility until the week he was moved to the hospital.

Keep checking in on your financial plan as your loved one's needs change. Be ready to make changes based on their health, finances, and any new help that becomes available. Stay in touch with the professionals helping you with the plan so you know about any new options or benefits that could help.

Summing It Up

The TL;DR is that financial planning is one of the most challenging aspects of caregiving. Many of us are not financial wizards to begin with. Financially planning for a long-term illness requires understanding short-term and long-term inflows and outflows of money for your loved one and yourself. It also requires consideration of employer benefits, insurance schemes, and the nonprofits around you. Your loved one's changing situation means finances are often in flux. Our family was lucky that my parents had been a dual-income household with health insurance and retirement savings. That savings quickly dwindled with supplemental therapies to try to keep dad's mind fresh and, later, to move him to memory care, which was astronomically costly and only private pay. Many options for professional caregiving support are only private pay. Insurance covers some health expenses, but never all of the psycho-therapeutic treatments you may want to try. Only you and your family can determine how to allocate the resources you have.

CHAPTER 9

Career Development

OVER THE COURSE OF MY DAD'S ILLNESS, EACH of his three kids finished terminal degrees in their fields and were on the hunt for jobs. We had interview processes, geographic changes, promotions, some successes, and some failures, including a firing. It was challenging to not have both parents available to be sounding boards during these times. We were still developing into "adults" and wanted to turn to our comfort people, but we quickly realized, as many before us have, that your parents will not be available forever. You have to make professional decisions for yourself.

I grew exponentially in terms of empathy and compassion and my understanding of medical processes and terminology during this period. That growth was an outcome of how I'd interacted with my family, other caregivers, other patients, and my dad. It was also, in part, an inspiration for this book.

I have two friends who epitomize the intersection of caregiving and professional development.

Sam's experience highlights how being a caregiver can really bleed into your professional life. She was pursuing a degree in psychotherapy, initially interested in working with young adults. As she watched her mother deal with Parkinson's, Sam found it easier to emotionally support her mom than her dad did. She took in stride the frustrations her mom expressed and the tension that seemed to build between her parents:

> I was able to detach from the situation enough to treat some interactions with Dad like a therapy session. I recognized he just needed someone to talk to, and he perceived that he didn't want to go to a professional therapist, because therapy was 'not for him,' so he talked to me instead. And talked. And talked. It built my counseling skills and my patience.

Sam now intends to work with older adults and caregivers. For her, caregiving support actually shifted her career path.

My friend Liz's career path was shaped by her mother's Alzheimer's diagnosis:

> I found myself a mother of two small children, just thirty years old, swept into the role of being responsible for my mother's life. I was on a course that no one else seemed to be on and I didn't have the first thing that felt like a road map with which to see it through. I couldn't turn to my friends for understanding, because no one else's parents had these same cognitive issues so young. It was isolating and there were days when I thought we were both losing our minds. The first few years of doctors' appointments, feeding grumpy babies in waiting rooms, an understandably scared mother, took their toll on me. I was having trouble processing these abrupt changes in my mom with whom I'd always been so close. On top of that, I knew she felt guilty for being what she felt was a burden on me and that maybe broke my heart worst of all. I saw the need to start a nonprofit that focused solely on the needs of caregivers.

Liz is now the founder of Mind What Matters, a nonprofit that gives cash grants to caregivers supporting a loved one with a neurologic impairment like Alzheimer's, Parkinson's, or ALS. She has become a local advocate for caregivers.

Sam and Liz may be extreme examples. Their caregiving experiences defined their professional trajectories. The relationship between your own caregiving experience and your career may be much more fluid.

Working and Caregiving

Reality for some caregivers can be very stark. The schedule and financial burden of caregiving causes them to leave the workforce entirely. Caregivers, especially female caregivers, tend to share the majority of child-rearing responsibilities even when working full time. Women are also more likely to become caregivers to their loved ones.[12, 13, 14] In some studies, researchers estimate that women make up 80 percent of the informal care workforce. This is not to say that men do not play a role in caregiving, but they tend to contribute to caregiving in other ways, and spend less time doing it. Men are more likely to suggest paying for outside help than contributing time themselves (the same is true with childcare).[15] Women are more likely to leave the paid labor force to become unpaid caregivers, leaving behind money and other financial and social resources. This can reduce their ability to balance things at home. It may mean more time for caregiving, but it can also mean an overwhelming burden of emotional grief and social isolation.

I met Maya in an online support group. She was a software engineer at a tech start-up. She had moved to San Francisco after being a lifelong New Yorker and was navigating a new city, a new job, and a new relationship. She liked it all and had just bought her first home. Maya was super-passionate about her work and, as the third hire at her company, stood to benefit financially if she stuck with her job and the company was sold. Things changed for Maya when her mother was diagnosed with advanced-stage multiple sclerosis. Overnight, Maya found herself facing a daunting choice: continue to focus on her career or leave her job to care for her mom full-time. She felt these were her only options, given her family dynamics.

Maya could not shake an overwhelming sense of guilt when she was across the country and unable to help her mom:

> In Maya's words, there was a constant voice in my head telling me I was violating the golden rule. I was not treating my mom like I would want to be treated. It brought me back to every childhood lesson my mom had taught me. I just felt like I would not forgive myself for having the wrong priorities. So I moved back.

Maya's new role was more challenging than expected. Just four months after she moved back to her mother's house, Maya had to move her mom to a hospice. It was a gut punch. Her mom was dying, and Maya had given up her entire adult life to be with her. She felt lost and drained on so many levels.

> I had a moment of absolute shock. What had I done and what was I going to do? I needed to grieve my mom, but I had no outlets besides being a caretaker. I was effectively starting over in all aspects of my life. Work and my ambition had always been so important to me. I had not applied for a job in a couple of years. How was I going to explain myself? I felt unprofessional. I felt fear and failure. It was a lot. My advice to myself would have been to not leave the workforce entirely. But hindsight is 20/20.

Maya got through it and is able to talk about her journey with humor and grace, but her experience is a reminder that caregiving decisions will impact your own professional life.

Consider Your Existing Employment

If you currently have a paid job outside of being a caregiver, you may wonder how you can possibly keep that job and take on more responsibilities at home. It is daunting. Just like Maya, you may decide to ultimately leave the workforce. But before doing so, it is worth looking into company policies that may support you to keep your job while caregiving.

Ask yourself a couple of fundamental questions:

- What is my financial bottom line? Specifically, what are my financial needs both for caregiving and for my personal life? Will I be spending more on caregiving than I am making in my job?
- What is my professional goal? Do I want to keep working in this job? How does my current job set me up for my future (in terms of next job, retirement, or meeting financial needs)?
- If I need or want to keep working, what do I need from my employer to sustain my work productivity?
- What will make me happy and fulfill me personally, given the financial realities I am facing?

If you reached question three, chances are you (for now) hope to stay in your aid job. This likely means having to cope with caregiving and working. Depending on the type of employer you have, there may be employee assistance available. Most employers who offer health insurance and paid leave benefits will have other benefits you may not be aware of. You can seek a human resource representative or your manager to learn more.

Here are the steps to take:

- Research Company Policies. Familiarize yourself with the company's policies and any existing provisions for caregiver support. This can include a review of your benefits package as well as in-person requirements. A flexible work schedule may be of interest to you.
- Know Your State Laws. Identify how the state you are in sets paid family leave. Most states have at least a few days paid family leave for caregivers. Often people use these days for caring for children, but they can also be used for other forms of caregiving. Reasonable accommodations for caregivers may also be required. If you can demonstrate that your loved one is dependent on you for assistance, your employer may be required to make accommodations that you request.
- Identify the Benefits of a Change that You Need. If you are going to request a modified schedule, then clearly articulate the advantages of a flexible schedule for both you and the employer. Highlight how it can contribute to your productivity, work–life balance, and overall job satisfaction. Additionally, emphasize how it can positively impact your ability to meet work responsibilities effectively. A friend of mine, coping with caregiving, requested working from home twice a week, which ultimately made it so they did not have to leave work as often.
- Prepare a Proposal. Develop a well-thought-out proposal outlining your requested schedule and how it aligns with your job requirements. Consider different flexible options such as adjusting start or end times, compressed workweeks, or remote work arrangements. Be prepared to explain how you will ensure continued productivity and address any potential concerns.

- Schedule a Meeting. Request a meeting with your supervisor or the appropriate HR representative to discuss your request. This allows for a more detailed conversation and ensures that you have their undivided attention.
- Follow Up in Writing. After the meeting, send a follow-up email summarizing the key points discussed and any agreed-upon next steps. This ensures clarity and provides a written record of the conversation.
- Remember That Finding a Balance between Caregiving and a Career Is an Ongoing Process. Be flexible and adapt your approach as needed. It's essential to regularly reassess and make adjustments to ensure that both your caregiving responsibilities and career goals are being met. Seek support, practice self-care, and maintain open communication with both your employer and loved ones to create a supportive environment that allows you to pursue your career aspirations while providing care.

Beyond official policies that can support you, there may be intangible aspects of work life that are important. The average person spends 81,396 hours at work—the equivalent of more than nine years. "Americans are now more likely to make friends at work than any other way—including at school, in their neighborhood, at their place of worship, or even through existing friends," according to the Survey Center on American Life.[16] In addition to an income, a job provides socialization with colleagues, a separation from your home life (if you work in person), and alone time as you commute (parents of small children will know that leaving the house each day by yourself can feel like a fete). Just being able to say to a colleague, "last night was rough, had to go to the hospital with my parent," can be helpful to your state of mind.

When you are caregiving, your work life can expand your support system. Researchers at the University of Pennsylvania and

University of Minnesota not only confirmed that close friendships increase workplace productivity, they also found out why: friends are more committed, communicate better, and encourage each other.[17] The deep understanding, mutual respect, and emotional support that come from these relationships can be incredibly beneficial in challenging times. So think how you can rely on colleagues (and colleague friends) who may become part of your caregiving journey simply because you see each other so often. Not everyone will have close friends at work, but for those who do, use them as a resource. A supportive colleague can step in to cover for you in a pinch, maybe by handling some of your tasks, attending meetings on your behalf, or just ensuring that your absence isn't felt too hard. On a particularly important day at work, my sister had to meet our dad at the hospital. Her team of interns stepped in and, with her on the phone, got the job done. Was it perfect? No. But it got done.

Work friends can reduce your work-related stress and help you focus on your caretaking role without worrying about work falling behind. Sometimes, you might need someone to advocate for your needs within the workplace or fend off pesky questions from others when you are having a crap day. A good colleague familiar with your situation can foster a more understanding and accommodating work environment. If nothing else, on days when everything seems overwhelming, a good colleague can provide the encouragement and motivation you need.

Changing the Professional Path

Like Maya, some caregivers decide to leave the workforce. This may be due to the type of job or its location or an assessment of the income relative to the cost of hiring caregiving help. Leaving the workforce is not always a choice, but it doesn't have to be doom and gloom.

I met Sarah through a caregiver network. Her mom was already on disability due to a workplace injury a decade prior. Her dad had been the primary caregiver before he was diagnosed with dementia.

I decided to leave behind my salaried job overseas, with its amazing benefits, to transition into a minimum wage part-time job at home. It was a tough call, but being there for my dad was my top priority. While I haven't jumped back into the workforce just yet, I've managed to line up a few part-time gigs that understand my need for flexibility to accommodate my dad's needs. This setup allows me to work different hours and days each week, which is a lifesaver right now. Eventually, I hope to transition into a more substantial role with one of these employers, especially since they've expressed interest in bringing me on board in a bigger capacity. On the other hand, I'm actually enjoying the variety of part-time work and might just stick with it even after I'm able to return to a full-time position. I've come to terms with the fact that my old life might be a thing of the past. The energy level I had before feels like a distant memory, and I know that getting back into my former specialty won't be easy. But I'm pushing forward, embracing new opportunities, and reminding myself that we're all capable of adapting and creating a new path in life.

Sarah shows that it doesn't have to be all or nothing. A career change may be a better fit than leaving the workforce entirely. Max was in his mid-thirties when we met. He had finished an advanced degree and was still living at home with his mom. She had been diagnosed with dementia a year prior and had taken a turn. He had older siblings, but they were all attached to kids or spouses and had less flexibility. When our conversation turned to work, Max was candid:

My job's pretty flexible, which is great, but it really eats up all my focus. And ever since my mom's health took a turn for the worse, I just can't seem to keep my head in the game. I've even started putting on weight. Trying to think about switching to an easier role? But it's like I'm scared and too tired to try anything new. All my colleagues are landing awesome new jobs and I'm just here, running on empty. It's a constant battle, you know? Mom's getting worse, work's a pressure cooker, I'm trying to take care of her, dealing with sibling drama, and the endless doctor visits. I'm all over the place. I can't even think about filling out a job form without going blank. Part of me wants to just quit, but that means no paycheck. I also don't want to stay and underperform and get fired. And the office vibe doesn't help; they clearly prefer people without all the family stuff to handle.

Max felt he was too young to leave the workforce entirely, but knew he needed to switch jobs. While he had the skills to work remotely and in a less demanding role, the decision was temporarily overwhelming and paralyzing. Luckily, he was able to make a move and, so far, it's working.

Full-Time Caregiving

Becoming a full-time caregiver is in some ways the hardest job in the world. It's like caring for a child who is not going to learn and grow. In fact, quite the opposite. There is no break, no off switch. If you are a full-time caregiver, you are a rockstar. When you start thinking about life beyond caregiving, note that the skills you are learning as a caregiver are actually invaluable and transferable.

If you want to rebuild a résumé and reenter the workforce, it can be helpful to think about what those skills are and how to pitch them.

Try to identify generally the tasks you have performed as a caregiver, factor out the skills, the level of responsibility, and the problem-solving tools you've used. In writing a cover letter for a new job, equate your caregiving skills to those that you may have used in a former career and how the reinforcement of these skills through caregiving can benefit a potential employer in a more permanent career.

Some may perceive caregiving as a career negative, but you can demonstrate that you saw it as an opportunity to be with family and for personal and professional growth. An unusual approach perhaps, but honesty can be powerful, and skills are skills. You are adding things to your toolkit even if you did take a different route to acquire them.

Here are some ways you can leverage your caregiving experience when searching for a job.

- Highlight Transferable Skills. Caregiving involves a range of transferable skills that can be valuable in many professions. These may include strong communication and interpersonal skills, empathy, problem-solving abilities, time management, organization, flexibility, and the ability to work under pressure. Identify and showcase these skills on your résumé and during interviews.
- Emphasize Responsibility and Reliability. Caregiving often requires a high level of responsibility, dependability, and trustworthiness. Employers value candidates who demonstrate reliability and the ability to handle sensitive and challenging situations with professionalism. Provide specific examples of your dependability and accountability in your caregiving role.
- Showcase Teamwork and Collaboration. As a caregiver, you may have worked with a multidisciplinary team, including healthcare professionals, therapists, and family members. Highlight your experience collaborating with others and emphasize your ability to work effectively in a team-oriented environment.

- Adaptability and Problem-Solving. Caregivers frequently encounter unexpected situations and must be adaptable and resourceful in finding solutions. Emphasize your ability to adapt to changing circumstances, think on your feet, and problem-solve effectively.
- Volunteer or Gain Additional Qualifications. Consider volunteering in related fields or pursuing additional qualifications that complement your caregiving experience. This could include certifications in healthcare, first aid, or specialized training relevant to the job you're seeking. These credentials can enhance your résumé and demonstrate your commitment to professional growth. The Alzheimer's Association, for example, looks for people who have experience of the disease to be support group leaders. Organizations value experience, and jobs value organizations.
- Network and Make Connections. Utilize your existing network, including healthcare professionals, organizations, or support groups, to explore job opportunities. Networking can provide valuable insights, recommendations, and access to potential employers who appreciate the skills gained from caregiving. I know two friends who met in a support group and ultimately made job changes as a result of those relationships. You never know who you may connect with.

Personal Growth

Reflection is powerful. It allows us to see light in the tunnel or, at a minimum, to distract ourselves. It may be hard to reflect on everything you have learned or may learn as a caregiver, but I grew, and each of my siblings grew, as a result of our experiences. I learned a new patience that I now translate into parenting. My brother improved his communications and self-expression, sharing his opinions and feelings in order to make shared decisions. My sister grew in terms of emotional regulation and stress management.

Here is a list of skills that caregivers build. It is not exhaustive, but it will help you identify areas in which you've grown while providing effective care and support for a loved one:

- Communication Skills. Caregivers enhance their communication skills to effectively interact with their loved ones, healthcare professionals, and other members of the care team. This includes active listening, clear expression of needs and concerns, and the ability to provide information and instructions in a compassionate and empathetic manner.

- Empathy and Compassion. Caregivers cultivate these qualities, which are vital for understanding and responding to the emotions and needs of their loved ones. They help caregivers provide emotional support, comfort, and encouragement during challenging times.

- Problem-solving and Decision-making. In response to challenges, caregivers learn to assess situations, evaluate options, and make informed decisions about care, treatment, and daily routines. Caregivers often have to think on their feet and find creative solutions to unexpected situations.

- Time Management and Organization. Caregiving requires excellent time management and organizational skills. Caregivers learn to prioritize tasks, manage schedules, coordinate appointments, and ensure medications are taken on time. They develop strategies to balance caregiving responsibilities with other personal and professional commitments.

- Health Monitoring and Basic Medical Knowledge. Caregivers acquire knowledge about their loved one's health condition and gain basic medical knowledge relevant to their care. They learn to monitor vital signs, observe symptoms, administer medications, and follow prescribed treatment plans. Caregivers often become proficient in managing medical equipment and handling emergency situations.

- Patience and Flexibility. Caregivers learn to adapt to changing circumstances, handle unexpected situations, and adjust caregiving strategies as needed. Patience and flexibility are essential when dealing with the physical and emotional needs of their loved ones.
- Stress Management. To cope with the physical and emotional demands of their responsibilities, caregivers learn to recognize signs of stress, practice self-care, engage in relaxation techniques, and seek support when needed. Caregivers prioritize their own well-being to prevent burnout and maintain their ability to provide quality care.
- Advocacy and Navigation Skills. Caregivers often become advocates for their loved ones within the healthcare system. They learn to navigate complex healthcare systems, ask questions, seek second opinions, and ensure their loved ones receive appropriate care and services. Caregivers develop skills to effectively communicate and collaborate with healthcare professionals.
- Self-reflection and Self-awareness. Caregivers learn to recognize their own limits, strengths, and emotions, and actively address their own well-being. Self-reflection helps caregivers understand their own needs, seek support, and make adjustments to provide better care.
- Resourcefulness and Research Skills. Caregivers become good at finding relevant information, community resources, support services, and available programs. They learn to utilize online resources, connect with support networks, and seek out specialized information to better care for their loved ones.

These skills are developed and refined over time as caregivers gain experience, seek knowledge, and adapt to the needs of their loved ones. A loved one's loss can lead you to grow and acquire new capacities that are useful beyond your caregiving role. Many millennial caregivers, for example, will learn to advocate for a loved one who not long ago advocated for them.

Summing It Up

Working and caregiving are challenging. Being a full-time caregiver is an act of love, perseverance, and pain. No matter how you cut the pie, there is not enough to go around. The TL;DR is that there are many modes of work today, so put thought and effort into finding the balance of caregiving and employment that works best for you. My mom kept working throughout my dad's illness. She had worked her entire life, paying her way through higher education to become the foremost expert in a particular type of law. Some of her best friends were colleagues she had worked with for decades. Her professional life sustained her when her home life was falling apart. And financially, she needed the benefits from her employer. The decision for her was easier because she also had children who could be caregivers. The key is finding the balance between the professional and the personal that works for your circumstances.

CHAPTER 10

Coping with Grief and Loss

ERHAPS ONE OF THE MOST CHALLENGING PARTS of caregiving is trying to grieve a loss while taking care of a person who is physically still alive, but no longer the same.

It wasn't until my dad passed away that I was able to remember who he really was. So calm, he rarely let little things bother him. He didn't say much unless he had to, and when he gave his opinion, we all listened. Happy and carefree, he was content with who he was and who we were as kids. Grounded. Loving. All of these wonderful qualities were sucked up by a deteriorating health condition. His personality changed because his brain was impacted. At times he knew that was happening, and he was deeply depressed and angry. Eventually, he just wasn't present.

We had to cope with each stage of his decline, with whoever he was going to be that day. We had to hold on to moments that he was his old self and prepare for moments of unpredictability. It was hard. There was extensive chronic anxiety associated with not knowing what to expect or when to expect it.

Coping with the way your loved one is declining is not the only challenge. You also have to cope with the judgment of others. There is a general misunderstanding among salespeople, servers, or folks on the street when they encounter a person who might look fine but whose brain is not working. My mom and sister took my dad to his favorite ice cream place. When he got to the counter, he couldn't get the words out to order a coffee frappe, his favorite treat. As he stared blankly at the person behind the counter, she became impatient. "*Sir?*" My mom tried to guide him without answering for him and diminishing his autonomy. "Dan, a frappe?" She said to the worker, "just a second." The worker got frustrated and asked him to step aside. By then, my dad was sullen, frustrated by his demoralizing limits. My mom asked my sister to take him to the car. She ordered the coffee frappe and pointedly said to the counter worker, "You wouldn't realize this, but he has Alzheimer's. He is not being indecisive. He can't get it out." It was bittersweet ice cream that night. For everyone.

These sorts of moments became commonplace when our family went out. Eventually, we did the ordering for the table and Dad ate what came. Later, we rarely went out to eat. It was too challenging. We felt lucky Dad had a dentist who understood his condition and treated him with kindness. One day, the dentist had a new staffer in the office who berated dad regarding his dental hygiene and asked questions related to his medications that he couldn't recall. When the dentist entered the room, he kindly apologized to Dad. He later told us he would work with his staff person.

In addition to your loved one's decline, you'll have to cope with changing family dynamics. For me, this involved my siblings and my mom. It was hard to celebrate big events in my life, like the birth of my second child, because my parents weren't there in the same way as they had been for my first child. I felt shortchanged. Of course, I am lucky they were there at all, but this feeling of "it's not the same" lingers. My friend Mae summed it up best: it's the loss of "what was" that really gets you. It shatters a stability that you've come to rely on, and figuring out how to put the family pieces back together can be nearly impossible. Some families do not recover from the loss and stress associated with the decline of a loved one.

The Toll of Caregiving

Caregiving takes an immense toll on caregivers. This is true for both spousal caregivers and children who take on caregiving rolls. Research has shown that individuals whose loved ones are facing a serious illness often experience higher levels of psychological distress, including symptoms of anxiety and depression. Researchers have found that adult children caring for a loved one with a serious illness have higher rates of depressive symptoms compared to those not in a caregiving role. The emotional toll of a loved one's illness may even have lasting effects on mental health. A report by the National Alliance for Caregiving and AARP found that caregivers of parents or parents-in-law with chronic conditions or disabilities are more likely to experience elevated stress, depression, and burnout compared to non-caregivers. In cases where a parent's illness is terminal, the emotional toll extends beyond the illness itself to the process of grieving and coping with the loss. The bereavement experience can vary widely, but studies have shown that losing a parent can lead to prolonged grief, feelings of emptiness, and a range of emotional challenges.

It is difficult to prepare yourself emotionally for a loved one's illness. The loss of a parent leaves you vulnerable. Many people are lucky enough to grow up with a stable parent or guardian, and the loss of that stability rocks your world. Parents (or guardians) are often figures of strength, care, and support. When they become ill, it can shatter their apparent invincibility. It can be emotionally jarring and difficult to acknowledge their vulnerability.

It can also create a reckoning with your own mortality. The illness of a loved one brings the realization that they are not going to live forever, and it confronts us with the reality that we won't, either. If you have not experienced a significant loss before, this can be a deeply distressing and an emotionally charged experience. There may also be tough conversations as your loved one copes with their own mortality and shares that struggle with you.

Beyond the reality of a potential death, there is the role reversal that comes into play. You may take on activities that your loved ones did for you as a child. Jake told me how unnerving it was to help his dad, a former high-school football coach and a really macho guy, out of the shower—he suddenly was a vulnerable, almost baby-like creature. The first time it happened, Jake fell apart. After his dad was dry, he went to his parent's spare bedroom and cried. This transition disrupts established dynamics and requires adjustment to new responsibilities and expectations.

Decline can bring with it a level of uncertainty you have never experienced before. The ultimate outcome may be obvious, but the timing and path to get there may be highly unpredictable. On top of this, seeing anyone you care about suffer is painful. Seeing it day in and day out can be scarring. In one unforgettable moment for our family, Dad simply laid down on the floor sobbing like a child. He was trapped in his body and mind, and there was nothing we could do for him.

Anticipatory Grief

Anticipatory grief is the deep sadness and emotional pain you feel when you know that a loved one is going to die, often because of a terminal illness or an incurable condition. It is a profound and complex process, first described over forty years ago by psychologist Pauline Boss. Often referred to as "ambiguous loss," it comes when the person you love is still physically present, but their personality, memories, and abilities are changing.

Anticipatory grief can be as taxing as any other form of loss. The anticipation of someone dying can be incredibly overwhelming because you know you're losing them, and yet you still have to go about life as if nothing has changed. This kind of grief can bring a lot of emotions, including sadness, anger, and anxiety. Sadness for the pain that your loved one is feeling. Anger for the changes to your own life that you are dealing with as a caregiver. Anxiety for what is to come and the financial toll that this disease is taking. There may even be a shameful, guilt-inducing hope that the loved one will pass and their suffering end.

The Effects of Grief

Physically, anticipatory grief (or any form of grief) can be exhausting. You might feel tired all the time, have trouble sleeping, or lose your appetite. It can feel like being depressed. My friend Emily had so much anxiety while caring for her dad, thinking about how he was doing and what might happen while she slept, that she could only sleep in thirty-minute spurts. It wasn't until she saw her own doctor for chronic migraines that she realized her lack of sleep was taking such a toll. She eventually had to get on medication to reset her circadian rhythms. Her dad ultimately had to move to a long-term care facility.

Many of these psychosomatic symptoms occur because your body is responding to the stress and emotional weight of knowing what's coming. You might also find it hard to focus on work or social

activities because your mind is constantly on your loved one and
the impending loss. You may start to pull away from others, feeling
isolated because you're dealing with such heavy emotions. This kind
of grief can also be isolating. You might feel like you're mourning
alone, as others may not fully understand the pain of losing someone
"a little bit at a time." It gets pretty challenging to constantly describe
to someone else what day-to-day life is like." It can also be emotionally exhausting because you are constantly adjusting to new realities
and what is now "normal."

For Liz, the hardest time was the holidays. Her mom was living with her, and they had always cooked for Christmas and
Thanksgiving together. They loved it. All of Liz's kids were involved.
Once Liz's mom had to move to a long-term care facility, the life
drained from those holidays. What once had been the happiest time
became the hardest. The hole was so big; it was hard for Liz to get out
of bed on those days. It took her two years to be able to cook again
on Thanksgiving, and she had to change the menu. The pain lingers.

One of the hardest aspects of anticipatory grief is its ongoing
nature. Unlike the grief that follows a death, this version doesn't have
a clear endpoint. Every time you notice a new change, it can feel
like a fresh loss. It can also be emotionally exhausting because you
are constantly adjusting to new realities and what is now "normal"

Kate's dad was an amazing storyteller. He would talk about
the time he went running with the bulls in Spain. His lead-up to the
run would last for ten minutes, and he built such anticipation you
couldn't wait to hear what happened next. The climax of the story
came when you realized that he'd watched the running of the bulls
from a balcony. When Kate went to visit him and he could no longer
tell that story, it took all of her strength to not run out in a puddle
of tears. She thought about that story for months. Why had she
not recorded him telling it? These moments can be heartbreaking
because you're not just losing a person to a disease—you're losing

the shared memories, the conversations, and the connection you once had.

However natural a reaction, it's important to recognize the feelings that accompany anticipatory grief and find ways to cope, whether by talking to friends, joining a support group, or seeking counseling. It's important to acknowledge the pain, allow yourself to grieve each loss as it comes, and find ways to cherish the moments of connection that remain.

Death Planning

Most families have trouble talking about death, however inevitable. But planning for a death can help alleviate some of the burdens and uncertainties associated with the decline of your loved one.

Here are some steps to consider when planning for a death:

- Identify Wishes. As early as possible, have open and honest conversations with your loved ones about end-of-life preferences and wishes. This should include topics like how they want to be buried (or cremated); what sort of end-of-life service they may want, such as a funeral or memorial service; if they would like to be an organ donor; and any specific requests that they may have. It's important to clearly communicate and ensure you are aware of your loved ones' wishes. These conversations may be more difficult for some than others. However, nearly everyone who I have talked to had an easier time after their loved one passed if they had the conversations ahead of time. We knew our dad wanted to be cremated. We knew he hated formality, so we had a memorial for him on a golf course. We joked there needed to be a ceremonial club toss on the fourteenth hole, since his game usually involved a tantrum somewhere on the back nine. The

event felt like a part of him we wanted to remember. Whatever
will feel meaningful for your family is a good place to start.

- Prepare Legal Documents. Consult with an attorney or estate
planner to prepare important legal documents, such as a will,
living will, healthcare proxy (or medical power of attorney), and
durable power of attorney. We mentioned these in the planning chapter (Chapter 3). These documents outline preferences
regarding medical decisions, asset distribution, and who will
act on your behalf in various situations. It is critical to choose
a trusted individual to serve as the executor or personal representative who will handle affairs after your loved one passes. If
you have partnered with loved ones, and one of them is ailing
but the other is of sound mind, then it may be the spouse,
but it does not have to be. Often, there is a legal representative who serves to formally execute a will. Ensure that whoever
is in charge is aware of their role and has access to important
documents, financial information, and passwords. If you are the
executor, be prepared.

- Review Life Insurance and Financial Accounts. Not everyone
has life insurance. Life insurance would likely have been taken
out at an earlier point in life when your loved one was planning
for the future and preparing for their death. There are two types
of life insurance: whole life insurance and term life insurance.
Whole life insurance is a policy that lasts for the person's whole
life and is paid out upon a person's death. Term life insurance
is a policy that has a fixed term or a fixed number of years for
which it is valid. A person may take out term life insurance until
they are age seventy, because they want the policy in case they
die at an earlier age when their family would have been more
dependent on their income. Find out if your loved one has life
insurance, and ensure life insurance policies are up to date and
that beneficiaries are named appropriately. It is also helpful to

have an inventory of financial accounts, investments, and assets, and ensure all necessary information is easily accessible to the executor.

- Communicate with Healthcare Providers. It may not always be obvious when the end is coming. Discuss pain management options and end-of-life care preferences, and explore hospice or palliative care services if appropriate. Is your priority for your loved one to simply be comfortable? Do you want any medical intervention possible? Do you have a do not resuscitate order if they go into cardiac arrest? These are all critical things to discuss with a healthcare provider. When your loved one has been deemed to be near the end of life, communicate their wishes with your healthcare providers. These moments creep up fast. Our dad was in hospital when we heard he needed to begin hospice care. Hospice care refers to a palliative state of care where the approach is to minimize pain, but not take any action to sustain life. When that call came, the facility believed he had approximately six months to live. Two days later, they called and said they believed he had two weeks to live. Three days later, the hospital called and said they believed he would die within twenty-four hours. From the time of that last call, he lived less than eight hours. It was a gut punch and a critical reminder that life will continue to surprise you.

- Identify a Funeral Home. In order for your loved one to leave the hospital or medical facility where they die, you have to identify a funeral home and have it come to get your loved one's body. If your loved one dies at home, you can call emergency services, and they will likely come to confirm the cause of death. It can be really helpful to have a funeral home or mortician in mind so that you are prepared. The moments after death are incredibly emotional and draining, and very quickly there are an overwhelming number of things to do. Consider creating an end-of-life plan that includes important information such as preferred funeral home, burial or cremation preferences, desired funeral or memorial service arrangements, and any specific requests for rituals or celebrations of life.

• Seek Emotional Support. It may be obvious from the tenor of this chapter, but it is critical to seek support for yourself. Support can look different for different people. Find what works for you, but recognize that your experience is likely going to change who you are. Reach out to a counselor, support group, or religious/spiritual leader to help you navigate the emotional aspects of planning for death. It can be beyond critical to have a supportive network during this time.

Loss

Coping with the loss of a loved one for whom you were the caregiver can be challenging and complex. Even if you are expecting the loss, and maybe hoping for the pain to end, the actual death will hit you hard. I thought I would be "ready" and yet for weeks and even months, the world felt surreal once the end had come.

Allow yourself to grieve and recognize that it is normal and healthy to experience a wide range of emotions, including sadness, anger, guilt, and confusion. You have just been through a life-changing experience. Now there will be a combination of relief, guilt, pain, and sadness. For many caregivers I have talked to, there is a sense of relief that comes with death, which is rarely discussed openly. There is a weight lifted by no longer watching your loved one suffer, and knowing you can now remember the easier times rather than the painful moments. As a caregiver, your life is now open in a fashion that you likely have not experienced in years. Give yourself permission to grieve and process your feelings at your own pace.

COPING WITH GRIEF AND LOSS   135

Now is a great time to seek additional support, either from your existing network or from new sources. Reach out to friends, family, or support groups who can provide understanding, empathy, and a safe space for you to express your emotions. Consider joining a bereavement group specifically for individuals who have been caregivers. It is critical to find healthy ways to express and process your emotions. This might involve talking to a trusted friend or therapist, writing in a journal, engaging in creative outlets like art or music, or practicing relaxation techniques such as deep breathing or meditation. If you find that your grief is overwhelming or interfering with your daily functioning, consider seeking support from a mental health professional. They can provide guidance and coping strategies, and help you navigate the complexities of grief. Healing takes time, and the grieving process is unique for everyone. Be patient with yourself, and allow yourself to heal in your own way and at your own pace.

Summing It Up

This chapter is heavy. The TL;DR is that coping with inevitable death while living is one of the hardest things to do. When loss first happens, you are like a wrecked ship, drowning in the water around you; as time goes by, the tides change and ebb and flow, and it gets easier to tolerate the water around you. It took several months for my overwhelming sense of loss to ease. The feelings still come, sometimes powerful enough to take my breath away, but in smaller moments. One of my favorite expressions has been that "grief comes in waves." Sometimes it sneaks up and takes your breath away.

I try to find ways to keep my dad's memory alive on a regular basis. Sometimes it happens spontaneously, like when I find myself thinking to text him when I am able to beat traffic or am excessively pissed off at one of my kids. For whatever is meaningful to you, find ways to honor and remember your loved one. This could involve creating a memory box, listening to their favorite songs, telling stories about them, or eating their favorite foods. We often eat strawberry shortcake and other desserts Dad loved. When our family gets together, we take out his collection of hats and encourage all of the grandchildren to try them on. My older son calls them "Papa's magician hats" (there are Charlie-Chaplin-style black-cloth bucket hats involved). Lean in to all of those iPhone photos you have, make a shared album, watch videos, do what you need to do to remember, and keep living.

Time will make things easier. It will not change the experience of growth and grief that you are experiencing.

Long-Term Illness Care Planning Template

Patient Information:

- Name:
- Date of Birth:
- Address:
- Phone Number:
- Emergency Contact:
- Primary Care Physician:
- Diagnosis:
- Current Medications:
- Allergies:

Goals of Care:

1. Identify the patient's goals, preferences, and values regarding their care.

2. Discuss the desired level of medical intervention, quality of life, and end-of-life preferences.
3. Ensure that the care plan aligns with the patient's goals and wishes.

Medical Team:

1. List all healthcare providers involved in the patient's care, including primary care physician, specialists, therapists, and caregivers.
2. Include contact information for each member of the medical team.

Treatment Plan:

1. Document the current treatment regimen, including medications, therapies, and medical procedures.
2. Review the effectiveness of treatments and discuss any changes or adjustments needed.
3. Coordinate care between different providers to ensure continuity and integration of services.

Symptom Management:

1. Identify common symptoms associated with the long-term illness and strategies for managing them.
2. Discuss pain management, symptom relief, and palliative care options.
3. Provide education and resources for caregivers on symptom recognition and management.

Nutrition and Hydration:

1. Assess the patient's nutritional needs and dietary preferences.
2. Develop a nutrition plan that supports the patient's overall health and well-being.
3. Monitor hydration status and provide recommendations for fluid intake.

Mobility and Activities of Daily Living (ADLs):

1. Evaluate the patient's mobility status and functional abilities.
2. Develop strategies to optimize independence in ADLs, such as bathing, dressing, and toileting.
3. Recommend assistive devices or modifications to the home environment as needed.

Emotional and Psychosocial Support:

1. Address the patient's emotional and psychosocial needs, including coping with stress, anxiety, and depression.
2. Offer counseling, support groups, or other mental health services to promote emotional well-being.
3. Provide resources and referrals for caregiver support and respite care.

Financial and Legal Planning:

1. Review the patient's financial situation, and discuss potential challenges related to the cost of care.

2. Assist with financial planning, insurance coverage, and access to financial assistance programs.
3. Address legal matters such as advance directives, powers of attorney, and estate planning.

Caregiver Support:

1. Assess the needs of caregivers and provide education, training, and resources to support their role.
2. Offer respite care options and connect caregivers with support groups or counseling services.
3. Develop a plan for backup caregivers in case of emergencies or caregiver burnout.

Follow-Up and Monitoring:

1. Schedule regular follow-up appointments to monitor the patient's progress and adjust the care plan as needed.
2. Coordinate communication between healthcare providers to ensure continuity of care.
3. Provide ongoing support and guidance to the patient and their caregivers throughout the illness journey.

Emergency Plan:

1. Develop a plan for managing medical emergencies, including instructions for contacting healthcare providers and accessing emergency services.
2. Ensure that caregivers are familiar with emergency procedures and have access to important medical information.
3. Review the emergency plan regularly and update as needed.

Notes and Additional Information:

- Document any additional information or considerations relevant to the patient's care plan.

- Encourage open communication and collaboration between the patient, caregivers, and healthcare providers.

- Reassess and update the care plan regularly to address changing needs and circumstances.

This template serves as a comprehensive guide for developing a care plan for individuals with long-term illnesses, promoting patient-centered care, collaboration among healthcare providers, and support for patients and their caregivers throughout the illness journey.

APPENDIX 2

Re-evaluation Care Planning Template

Date:

Parent's Information

Name: Age:

Diagnosis:

Current living situation:

Health Status:

Physical abilities: [Note any difficulties with mobility, driving, cooking, dressing, bathing, using the bathroom, hearing, vision, etc.]

Cognitive status: [Note any concerns with memory, problem-solving, attention, or confusion]

Medications: [List current medications and dosage schedule]

Symptoms: [List any concerning symptoms or changes]

Doctors: [List medical providers and contact info]

Social/Lifestyle Considerations

Social engagement: [Note any changes in social activities or relationships]

Community mobility: [Assess ability to access services, transportation, etc.]

Home safety risks: [Check for fall hazards, cleanliness, accessibility]

Caregiver support: [Identify current formal or informal caregivers]

Recommendations

[List any recommended actions, such as]:

- Home health assistance
- Additional medical follow-up
- Home modifications
- Assistive equipment
- Community programs
- Support groups
- Legal assistance

Next Steps

[Outline specific next steps with responsibility and timeframe, such as the following]:

1. Schedule doctor appointment for new symptoms (Who will do it and when)
2. Arrange home safety assessment (Who will do it and when)
3. Research adult day programs (Who will do it and when)

This template allows family members to collaborate and document concerns, needs, and plans to best support their parent's health and well-being. The recommendations and next steps sections prompt the creation of an action plan.

The CALMER Steps to Balancing Caregiving Responsibility

STEP 1: **Clarify** what you know (medically)

The first step is to take stock of what you know about the condition you are facing. Consult with your loved one's clinical care team. What is the prognosis? What is the timeline? Is there a "typical" case? Do you have access to a clinical coordinator? Make these clarifications regular. Never be afraid to ask questions.

STEP 2: **Acknowledge** what you don't know

Even with the best medical team, most long-term illnesses come with a lot of unknowns. In our experience, it is critical to recognize that there will often not be clear answers to your most pressing questions. It may be challenging to know how quickly the illness will progress and what support you will need. Write down your open questions. Revisit them.

STEP 3: **List** your priorities

There are probably an endless number of things you feel like you need to do, so having priorities can help you to organize where to go next. For some families, the first priority is identifying a support system: who will help with care, cooking, transportation, etc. For others, the first priority is social and emotional help.

STEP 4: **Make** small steps

Figuring out how to achieve your priorities is perhaps the hardest part. Oftentimes you are overwhelmed and charting new territory. We suggest starting small. Identify who you already know and may be available to help once a week. Start ordering groceries instead of needing to make a daily run. Ask your local pharmacy for pill packs so you can stay organized. Sound overwhelming? Small things are in *your* control, even when the big stuff is not.

STEP 5: **Encourage** support

We know that you may not have listed finding support as a top priority, but it can be absolutely critical. That is why we offer unlimited support groups, on-demand, and access to a peer supporter through our platform. In your daily life, allow others to help you. Coping with illness is not a short-term deal. Taking breaks can save your own health. So is finding a new routine that includes self-care alongside caregiving responsibilities.

STEP 6: **Re-evaluate** consistently

Long-term illness is dynamic. Prognoses can change. You may notice differences in your loved one more quickly than you thought you would. You may also realize that what you thought would work for your family is no longer the case.

It's critical to re-evaluate and follow the CALMER steps as things move.

Financial Budget Worksheet

Category	Estimated Credits/ Inflows ($)	Estimated Debits/ Outflows ($)	Notes	Total ($)
1. Income:				
Salary or wages from employment				
Caregiver support or stipend, if applicable				
Benefits or allowances from government programs, if eligible				
Any additional sources of income (e.g., rental income, investments)				
2. Fixed Expenses:				
Rent or mortgage payment				
Utilities (electricity, water, gas)				
Internet and phone bills				
Health insurance premiums				

Category	Estimated Credits/ Inflows ($)	Estimated Debits/ Outflows ($)	Notes	Total ($)
Car payments or transportation expenses				
Loan repayments (student loans, personal loans, etc.)				
Childcare or education expenses, if applicable				
3. Variable Expenses:				
Groceries and household supplies				
Personal care items (toiletries, medications, etc.)				
Transportation (fuel, public transportation, maintenance)				
Medical expenses (prescriptions, copayments, deductibles)				
Caregiving supplies (incontinence products, medical equipment, etc.)				
Entertainment and leisure activities				
Dining out or meals on the go				
Miscellaneous expenses (gifts, subscriptions, hobbies)				
4. Caregiving Expenses:				
Medical supplies or equipment not covered by insurance				
Prescription medications				
Home modifications or accessibility adaptations				

Category	Estimated Credits/ Inflows ($)	Estimated Debits/ Outflows ($)	Notes	Total ($)
Professional caregiving services or respite care, if needed				
Co-payments or deductibles for medical appointments or treatments				
Other specific caregiving-related expenses				
5. Savings and Emergency Fund:				
Allocate a portion of your income toward savings for emergencies and future needs. Aim to save at least 10-15% of your income, if possible.				
6. Debt Repayment:				
If you have any outstanding debts, allocate a portion of your income toward debt repayment. Consider prioritizing high-interest debts first.				
7. Miscellaneous Expenses:				
Allocate a small portion of your budget for unexpected expenses or miscellaneous needs that may arise.				

NOTES

1 https://www.nia.nih.gov/health/what-are-signs-alzheimers-disease
2 https://jamanetwork.com/journals/jamaneurology/fullarticle/2781919.
3 https://www.ncbi.nlm.nih.gov/books/NBK543712/#
4 https://doi.org/10.26419/ppi.00103.013
5 Gutterman, A.S., "Caregiving and Families," 2023. Available at SSRN 4610245.
6 Peterson, N., et al., "Stress and Supportive Care Needs of Millennial Caregivers: A Qualitative Analysis," 2021. https://doi.org/10.1177/01939459211056689
7 Arensberg, L.C., Kalender-Rich, J., Lee, J., and Gibson, CA., "Millennials Seeking Healthcare: Examining the Degree to Which Patients Utilize Online Resources." *Kansas Journal of Medicine*, 2022;15:347.
8 Lau, J.S., Adams, S.H., Boscardin, W.J., and Irwin Jr C.E., "Young Adults' Health Care Utilization and Expenditures Prior to the Affordable Care Act." *Journal of Adolescent Health*, 2014 Jun 1;54(6):663–71.
9 Fronstin, P., "Consumer Engagement in Health Care among Millennials, Baby Boomers, and Generation X: Findings from the 2017 Consumer Engagement in Health Care Survey." EBRI Issue Brief, 2018 Mar 5(444).
10 Pohl, J., Kolodisner, J., and Coon, D., "Family Caregiver Social Connectedness: Technology Use Across Generations during the COVID-19 Pandemic." *Innovation in Aging*, 2022, 6(Supplement_1):101–101.
11 Primack, B.A. et al., Social Media Use and Perceived Social Isolation Among Young Adults in the US. *American Journal of Preventive Medicine*, 2017 Jul 1;53(1):1–8.
12 Lee, Y., and Tang, F., "More Caregiving, Less Working: Caregiving Roles and Gender Difference." *Journal of Applied Gerontology*, 2015, 34(4), 465–483.

13 Navaie-Waliser, M., Spriggs, A., and Feldman, P. H. "Informal Caregiving: Differential Experiences by Gender." *Medical Care*, 2002, 1249–1259.

14 Sharma, N., Chakrabarti, S., and Grover, S., "Gender Differences in Caregiving among Family – Caregivers of People with Mental Illnesses." *World Journal of Psychiatry*, 2016 Mar 22;6(1):7–17. https://doi.org/10.5498/wjp.v6.i1.7. PMID: 27014594; PMCID: PMC4804270.

15 https://www.pewresearch.org/social-trends/2017/03/23/gender-and-caregiving/

16 https://hbr.org/2022/10/the-power-of-work-friends

17 Jehn, K. A., and Shah, P. P., "Interpersonal Relationships and Task Performance: An Examination of Mediation Processes in Friendship and Acquaintance Groups." *Journal of Personality and Social Psychology*, 1997;72(4), 775–790. https://doi.org/10.1037/0022-3514.72.4.775